INTRODUCTION

The concept of the Blood Type Diet, popularized by Dr. Peter D'Adamo in his book "Eat Right for Your Type," has garnered attention for its assertion that an individual's blood type influences their dietary requirements. According to this theory, people with blood type O have distinct nutritional needs that are tailored to their genetic makeup. This introduction will delve into the characteristics of blood type O and explore the proposed role of diet in optimizing health for individuals with this blood type.

Blood type O is characterized by the presence of specific antigens on the surface of red blood cells. These antigens, namely A and B, are absent in blood type O, making it the universal donor for blood transfusions. Beyond its relevance in medical contexts, proponents of the Blood Type Diet claim that blood type O is associated with specific ancestral traits, linking individuals with this blood type to ancient hunter-gatherer societies.

The central premise of the Blood Type Diet is that blood type influences how the body reacts to different foods, impacting digestion, metabolism, and overall well-being. For those with blood type O, the recommended dietary approach aligns with what is often described as a "hunter" or "ancestral" diet. This diet emphasizes high-quality animal proteins, such as lean meat, fish, and poultry, on the assumption that individuals with blood type O have a digestive system optimized for protein consumption.

The diet suggests limiting or avoiding certain foods that proponents claim may be less compatible with blood type O. For instance, dairy products and grains containing gluten are often discouraged, as they are believed to be less consistent with the digestive characteristics associated with blood type O. In addition to specific food recommendations, the Blood Type Diet proposes that individuals with blood type O may benefit from engaging in certain types of exercise tailored to their supposed ancestral predispositions.

CHAPTER ONE

Definition of Blood Type O

Blood type O refers to one of the four main blood types in the ABO blood group system. In this system, blood is categorized based on the presence or absence of specific antigens on the surface of red blood cells. Blood type O individuals are characterized by the absence of both A and B antigens, making their blood type compatible as universal donors for blood transfusions. The defining factor for blood type O is the presence of anti-A and anti-B antibodies in the plasma.

Here's a breakdown of the critical components:

1. Antigens: Blood type O is distinguished by the absence of A and B antigens on the surface of red blood cells. Antigens are proteins or carbohydrates that trigger immune responses. In the case of blood type O, individuals do not have A or B antigens, but they have both anti-A and anti-B antibodies in their plasma.

2. Universal Donor: Blood type O is often referred to as the universal donor because individuals with type O blood can donate to individuals of any blood type (O, A, B, or AB) without causing an adverse immune reaction. This makes type O blood crucial in emergency situations when the recipient's blood type is unknown or when there is a shortage of a specific blood type.

3. Compatibility: Blood type O individuals can receive

blood only from donors with type O. This is due to the presence of anti-A and anti-B antibodies in their plasma, which would react with A or B antigens if introduced. However, type O-negative blood is often used in emergencies because it lacks both A and B antigens, minimizing the risk of adverse reactions.

4. Genetic Basis: Blood type is inherited from parents. The ABO blood group system is determined by the presence or absence of specific genes (IA, IB, and i). The combination of these genes inherited from each parent determines an individual's blood type. Blood type O individuals typically inherit two "i" genes.

Understanding blood types is crucial in various medical contexts, including blood transfusions, organ transplants, and pregnancy. It plays a significant role in determining donor-recipient compatibility and helps prevent immune reactions that could be harmful to the recipient. Blood type O, with its unique characteristics, plays a vital role in ensuring the availability of compatible blood for patients in need.

BLOOD TYPE O CHARACTERISTICS

A. Genetic and Anthropological Background:

1. Hunter-Gatherer Ancestry: Blood Type O is often associated with a hunter-gatherer ancestry, reflecting a historical perspective on human evolution. Proponents of this idea suggest that individuals with blood type O share genetic traits with early hunter-gatherer populations. These populations were characterized by a diet rich in animal proteins and a lifestyle that involved physical activity and adaptability to various environments.

2. Evolutionary Factors Influencing Blood Type O: The prevalence of blood type O in certain regions is believed to be influenced by evolutionary factors. Some theories propose that efficiently digesting animal proteins, a characteristic associated with blood type O, conferred a survival advantage in environments where plant-based food sources were scarce. Over time, these genetic traits became more prevalent in populations with a history of relying on hunting and animal-based diets.

B. Personality Traits Associated with Blood Type O:

1. Traits Commonly Attributed to "Hunters": Personality traits associated with blood type O are often described in terms of the characteristics of hunters. These traits

include a robust and self-reliant nature, adaptability, and a focus on goals. In this context, Hunters are considered decisive individuals who approach challenges with a practical and action-oriented mindset. The idea is that these traits reflect the adaptive qualities required for survival in hunter-gatherer societies.

2. Behavioral Tendencies Based on Blood Type: While the scientific validity of personality traits being directly linked to blood type is widely debated, some popular beliefs associate specific behavioral tendencies with blood type O. These include traits such as assertiveness, a competitive spirit, and a tendency to be outgoing. It's essential to approach these associations with caution, as personality is a complex and multifaceted aspect of human behavior influenced by various factors, including genetics, environment, and personal experiences.

BLOOD TYPE AND DISEASE SUSCEPTIBILITY

1. Overview of Studies Linking Blood Type to Specific Health Conditions: Research has explored potential links between blood type and susceptibility to specific health conditions over the years. While findings are often preliminary and subject to ongoing investigation, some associations have been observed. One of the most well-known connections involves the ABO blood group system and the risk of certain diseases. For example:

• Cardiovascular Disease: Some studies have suggested that individuals with blood type O may have a lower risk of cardiovascular diseases, while those with blood type A or AB might be at a higher risk. The mechanisms underlying these associations are not fully understood but may involve factors such as blood clotting tendencies.

• Blood Clotting Disorders: Blood type A has been associated with a higher risk of venous thromboembolism, a condition involving blood clot formation. Blood type O is linked to a potentially lower risk of blood clotting disorders.

• Infectious Diseases: There is ongoing research on the

relationship between blood type and susceptibility to certain infectious diseases. For example, some studies have explored the potential association between blood type and the risk of contracting certain viruses, such as norovirus and H. pylori infection.

1. Genetic Factors Influencing Susceptibility: The ABO blood group is determined by the presence or absence of specific antigens and antibodies, which are influenced by genetic factors. The genetic basis of blood type may contribute to variations in disease susceptibility. Key points to consider include:

• A and B Antigens: The presence or absence of A and B antigens on red blood cells is determined by the inheritance of specific genes (IA, IB, and i). These genes dictate the production of enzymes responsible for adding A or B antigens to the red blood cell surface. The combination of these genes inherited from each parent determines an individual's blood type.

• Immune Responses: The ABO blood group system also influences immune responses. Individuals with blood type A produce antibodies against type B antigens, and vice versa. Blood type O individuals produce antibodies against both A and B antigens. These immune responses may play a role in disease susceptibility, particularly in conditions involving immune-related mechanisms.

• Inflammatory Responses: The ABO blood group has been implicated in modulating inflammatory responses. Inflammatory processes are integral to the body's defense mechanisms, but dysregulation can contribute to various diseases. The specific ways in which blood type influences inflammatory pathways are areas of active research.

IMMUNE SYSTEM CHARACTERISTICS

1. Immune Response Variations in Blood Type O: The immune system, a complex network of cells and proteins, plays a crucial role in defending the body against infections and diseases. While individual immune responses are influenced by a myriad of factors, including genetics and environmental exposures, some studies have explored potential variations in resistant characteristics based on blood type, with a focus on Blood Type O.

• Antibody Production: Blood Type O individuals are known to produce antibodies against both A and B antigens, a characteristic not shared with individuals of other blood types. This unique feature may impact the immune response by influencing the body's ability to recognize and target specific pathogens.

• Inflammatory Responses: The ABO blood group system has been implicated in modulating inflammatory responses. Blood Type O individuals, in particular, may exhibit differences in inflammatory markers, potentially affecting the body's response to infections and inflammatory conditions. The specifics of these variations and their impact on overall immune function are areas of ongoing research.

• Blood Clotting and Immunity: Some studies suggest that blood type O individuals may have a lower risk of certain blood clotting disorders. This may be linked to immune-related factors, as blood clotting and immune responses are interconnected. Understanding these connections is vital in comprehending how blood type O may influence susceptibility to conditions involving immune dysregulation.

1. Impact on Susceptibility to Infections and Immune-Related Disorders: The relationship between blood type O and susceptibility to infections and immune-related disorders is a complex interplay of genetic, immunological, and environmental factors. While the scientific community continues to explore these connections, some observations have been made:

• Infectious Diseases: Studies have investigated whether blood type O individuals may have varying susceptibility to certain infections. For example, there is ongoing research on the potential associations between blood type and susceptibility to viruses such as norovirus, H. pylori, and certain strains of influenza. The mechanisms underlying these associations may involve interactions between viral antigens and blood group antigens.

• Autoimmune Disorders: Autoimmune disorders are complex and multifactorial, where the immune system mistakenly attacks the body's own tissues. While no direct causative link has been established between blood type and autoimmune diseases, there is interest in understanding how variations in immune responses associated with different blood types may influence the development or progression of autoimmune conditions.

• Blood Clotting Disorders: Blood clotting is another facet

of immune function, and variations in blood clotting mechanisms have been associated with different blood types. Blood type O individuals may have a lower risk of certain blood clotting disorders, which could have implications for conditions related to vascular health.

AN OVERVIEW OF DIET PHILOSOPHY

Diet philosophy encompasses the principles and beliefs that guide an individual's or a community's approach to food and nutrition. It goes beyond the mere selection of foods for sustenance and delves into the broader concepts of health, well-being, and the relationship between food and various aspects of life. Different diet philosophies often reflect cultural, ethical, health-centric, or even spiritual values. Here are the major components that contribute to diet philosophy:

1. Nutritional Approach: Diet philosophy starts with a fundamental consideration of dietary principles. This includes understanding macronutrients (carbohydrates, proteins, and fats), micronutrients (vitamins and minerals), and their role in maintaining optimal health. Some diet philosophies may emphasize specific ratios of macronutrients or focus on whole, minimally processed foods.

2. Cultural and Ethical Dimensions: Cultural and ethical beliefs heavily influence diet philosophy. Cultural practices, traditions, and values often dictate dietary choices. Additionally, ethical considerations, such as environmental sustainability, animal welfare, and fair trade, can shape nutritional preferences. Veganism,

vegetarianism, and various sustainable food movements are examples of diet philosophies grounded in cultural and ethical principles.

3. Holistic Health: Many diet philosophies adopt a holistic approach to health, recognizing the interconnectedness of physical, mental, and emotional well-being. They may consider factors beyond nutrition, such as stress management, sleep, and physical activity. The goal is to promote overall health and prevent disease rather than merely addressing nutritional needs in isolation.

4. Personalized Nutrition: Acknowledging that individuals have unique nutritional requirements, customized nutrition is gaining prominence in diet philosophy. This approach considers factors such as age, gender, genetics, health status, and personal preferences to tailor dietary recommendations for optimal well-being. It moves away from a one-size-fits-all mentality, recognizing the diversity of nutritional needs.

5. Mindful Eating: Mindful eating is a diet philosophy that encourages a present and intentional approach to eating. It involves paying attention to hunger and fullness cues, savoring flavors, and being conscious of the eating experience. This philosophy aims to foster a healthier relationship with food, promoting mindful consumption and preventing overeating.

6. Functional Foods and Nutraceuticals: Some diet philosophies emphasize the role of functional foods and nutraceuticals—foods with potential health benefits beyond essential nutrition. This may include foods rich in antioxidants, phytochemicals, or specific nutrients believed to have therapeutic properties. The focus is on using food as a preventive and restorative tool.

7. Intermittent Fasting and Time-Restricted Eating: Time-restricted eating and intermittent fasting have gained popularity as diet philosophies that prescribe specific periods of eating and fasting. These approaches are believed to have various health benefits, including improved metabolic health and weight management. They highlight not only what but also when to eat for optimal health.

8. Anti-Inflammatory Diets: Recognizing the role of inflammation in various chronic diseases, some diet philosophies center around anti-inflammatory principles. These diets emphasize foods that may reduce inflammation, such as fruits, vegetables, fatty fish, and nuts, while limiting inflammatory triggers like processed foods and sugar.

FUNDAMENTAL PRINCIPLES OF THE BLOOD TYPE O DIET

1. High Protein Intake: Blood Type O individuals are often advised to follow a high-protein diet, with an emphasis on lean sources. This dietary recommendation is rooted in the belief that individuals with blood type O may have a digestive system optimized for the efficient metabolism of animal proteins. Recommended sources include:

• Lean Meat: Lean beef, lamb, and venison cuts are often suggested.

• Poultry: Chicken and turkey are considered suitable protein sources.

• Fish: Fatty fish like salmon, cod, and mackerel are recommended for their omega-3 fatty acids.

1. Limited Grains: The Blood Type O diet typically recommends limited consumption of grains, with a particular emphasis on avoiding certain types of grains, especially those containing gluten. The rationale is based on the idea that individuals with blood type O may have a lower tolerance for specific grain proteins.

Recommendations include:

• Avoidance of Wheat: Wheat and wheat-based products are often discouraged due to their gluten content.

• Focus on Rice and Quinoa: Rice and quinoa are often considered more compatible grain options for individuals with blood type O.

1. Dairy Considerations: Blood Type O individuals are advised to limit their intake of dairy products. The rationale is that some individuals with blood type O may be lactose intolerant or have difficulty digesting certain dairy proteins. Specific recommendations include:

• Limited Dairy: Restricting or moderating the consumption of dairy products such as milk, cheese, and yogurt.

• Emphasis on Certain Cheeses: If consumed, certain cheeses like feta or goat cheese may be recommended over others.

1. Beans and Legumes: The Blood Type O diet suggests moderation in consuming beans and legumes. While they are considered a good source of plant-based protein, certain types may be recommended in limited quantities or avoided altogether. Guidelines include:

• Limited Intake of Certain Beans: Adzuki beans, lentils, and black-eyed peas are often suggested in moderation.

• Avoidance of Certain Legumes: Beans like kidney beans and navy beans may be recommended to be avoided or consumed sparingly.

1. Vegetable Choices: The diet encourages the consumption of a variety of vegetables, with a focus on nutrient-dense and non-starchy options. Leafy greens

and certain vegetables are often recommended:

• Emphasis on Leafy Greens: Spinach, kale, and broccoli are often highlighted for their nutrient content.

• Recommended Vegetables: Other recommended vegetables may include Brussels sprouts, sweet potatoes, and pumpkins.

1. Fruits in the Diet: Fruits are generally considered a healthy component of the Blood Type O diet, but there are specific recommendations regarding the types and amounts to consume:

• Recommended Fruits: Berries, cherries, and plums are often suggested.

• Moderation of Certain Fruits: Fruits such as oranges and strawberries may be recommended in moderation.

1. Nuts and Seeds: Nuts and seeds are considered beneficial for Blood Type O individuals, providing healthy fats and protein. Specific guidelines include:

• Recommended Nuts: The diet often includes walnuts, pumpkin seeds, and almonds.

• Limitation of Peanuts: Peanuts may be limited due to concerns about lectin content.

ACKNOWLEDGMEN T OF INDIVIDUAL DIFFERENCES

1. Genetic Diversity within Blood Type Groups: It is essential to recognize that even within broad blood type categories such as A, B, AB, and O, considerable genetic diversity exists among individuals. The ABO blood group system, while categorizing individuals based on the presence or absence of A and B antigens, doesn't capture the full spectrum of genetic variation. Genetic diversity extends beyond blood type, including factors influencing metabolism, nutrient absorption, and response to specific dietary components.

• Rh Factor: The ABO blood type system doesn't account for the Rh factor (positive or negative), adding another layer of genetic diversity within each blood type group.

• Genetic Polymorphisms: Variations in specific genes, known as genetic polymorphisms, contribute to individual differences in how the body processes nutrients. For example, genetic variations can influence responses to dietary fats, carbohydrates, and micronutrients.

1. Importance of Personalized Nutrition: Acknowledging

individual differences, including genetic diversity, emphasizes the importance of personalized nutrition. This approach recognizes that a one-size-fits-all dietary recommendation may only be optimal for some. Several factors contribute to the need for customized nutrition:

• Metabolic Variability: Individuals exhibit variability in metabolic rates, nutrient requirements, and how their bodies respond to different types and amounts of food. Personalized nutrition considers these metabolic differences.

• Health Conditions and Risks: Personalized nutrition takes into account individual health conditions, risk factors, and specific nutritional needs. Conditions such as diabetes, cardiovascular disease, and food allergies necessitate tailored dietary approaches.

• Lifestyle and Preferences: Personalized nutrition also considers individual lifestyles, cultural preferences, and dietary habits. Adapting dietary recommendations to align with an individual's lifestyle increases the likelihood of adherence to nutritional guidelines.

• Nutrigenomics and Nutrigenetics: These emerging fields explore the relationship between genetics and nutrition. Nutrigenomics examines how nutrients interact with genes, influencing health and disease. Nutrigenetics focuses on how genetic variations affect responses to diet. Integrating these principles into personalized nutrition allows for a more precise understanding of individual dietary needs.

• Microbiome Influence: The composition of the gut microbiome varies among individuals and can impact how the body processes certain nutrients. Personalized nutrition considers the role of the microbiome in optimizing health.

nutrition considers the role of the microbiome in optimizing health.

CHAPTER TWO

Lean Meats Recipes

Lemon Herb Grilled Chicken Breast Salad Bowl

Meal Description: This refreshing and light Grilled Lemon Herb Chicken Breast Salad Bowl perfectly balances flavors and textures. Tender grilled chicken breasts marinated in a zesty lemon herb dressing are served atop a bed of crisp mixed greens, cherry tomatoes, cucumber slices, and avocado. The dish is finished with a drizzle of the remaining marinade for a burst of citrusy goodness.

Ingredients: For the Lemon Herb Marinade:

• Two tablespoons of olive oil

• One tablespoon of fresh lemon juice

• One teaspoon of lemon zest

• Two cloves garlic, minced

• One teaspoon dried oregano

• One teaspoon of dried thyme

• Salt and black pepper to taste

For the Grilled Chicken:

• Two boneless, skinless chicken breasts

• Lemon slices for garnish (optional)

For the Salad Bowl:

• 4 cups mixed greens

• 1 cup cherry tomatoes, halved

• One cucumber, thinly sliced

• One avocado, sliced

Instructions:

1. Whisk together all the ingredients for the lemon herb marinade in a small bowl.

2. Place the chicken breasts in a resealable plastic bag and pour half of the marinade over them. Seal the bag, ensuring the chicken is well-coated. Marinate in the refrigerator for at least 30 minutes.

3. Preheat the grill to medium-high heat.

4. Remove the chicken from the marinade, allowing any excess to drip off. Grill the chicken for 6-8 minutes per side or until fully cooked with excellent grill marks. Baste the chicken with the remaining marinade during grilling.

5. While the chicken is grilling, prepare the salad bowl. Divide the mixed greens among serving bowls and top with cherry tomatoes, cucumber slices, and avocado.

6. Once the chicken is cooked, slice it into thin strips.

7. Arrange the grilled chicken on top of the salad bowls. Drizzle any remaining marinade over the chicken and salad.

8. Garnish with lemon slices if desired. Serve immediately and enjoy this delightful, low-calorie meal!

Nutrition Information (per serving): Calories: 240 Protein: 25g Carbohydrates: 10g Fat: 12g Saturated Fat: 2g Cholesterol: 60mg Sodium: 160mg Fiber: 5g Sugar: 2g

BAKED TURKEY MEATBALLS WITH ZUCCHINI NOODLES

Meal Description: This recipe brings together lean and flavorful baked turkey meatballs served over a bed of fresh zucchini noodles. The turkey meatballs are seasoned with a blend of herbs and spices, ensuring a burst of savory goodness in every bite. Paired with light and nutritious zucchini noodles, this dish is a delicious and satisfying low-carb alternative to traditional pasta.

Ingredients:

For the Turkey Meatballs:

• 1 pound ground turkey

• 1/2 cup breadcrumbs (whole wheat or gluten-free)

• 1/4 cup grated Parmesan cheese

• 1/4 cup finely chopped fresh parsley

• One egg

• Two cloves garlic, minced

• One teaspoon dried oregano

- One teaspoon of dried basil
- Salt and pepper to taste

For the Zucchini Noodles:

- Four medium-sized zucchini, spiralized
- One tablespoon of olive oil
- Salt and pepper to taste

For the Tomato Sauce:

- One can (14 ounces) crushed tomatoes
- Two cloves garlic, minced
- One teaspoon of dried Italian seasoning
- Salt and pepper to taste

For Garnish:

- Fresh basil leaves, chopped
- Grated Parmesan cheese

Instructions:

1. Preheat the oven to 400°F (200°C).

2. In a large mixing bowl, combine all the ingredients for the turkey meatballs - ground turkey, breadcrumbs, Parmesan cheese, parsley, egg, garlic, oregano, basil, salt, and pepper. Mix until well combined.

3. Shape the mixture into meatballs, approximately 1 to 1.5 inches in diameter, and place them on a baking sheet lined with parchment paper.

4. Bake the meatballs in the preheated oven for 20-25 minutes or until they are cooked through and browned on the outside.

5. While the meatballs are baking, prepare the zucchini

noodles. In a large skillet, heat olive oil over medium heat. Add the spiralized zucchini, salt, and pepper. Sauté for 3-5 minutes until the noodles are just tender. Remove from heat.

6. Combine the crushed tomatoes, minced garlic, Italian seasoning, salt, and pepper in a separate saucepan. Simmer over low heat for about 10 minutes to allow the flavors to meld.

7. Once the meatballs are done baking, place them on top of the zucchini noodles. Spoon the tomato sauce over the meatballs and noodles.

8. Garnish with chopped fresh basil and grated Parmesan cheese.

9. Serve immediately, and enjoy this healthy and flavorful baked turkey meatballs with zucchini noodles!

Nutrition Information (per serving): Calories: 320 Protein: 30g Carbohydrates: 15g Fat: 15g Saturated Fat: 4g Cholesterol: 110mg Sodium: 550mg Fiber: 4g Sugar: 7g

PAN-SEARED SALMON WITH DILL SAUCE

Meal Description: This recipe features succulent pan-seared salmon fillets drizzled with a vibrant dill sauce. The crispy skin on the salmon contrasts perfectly with the flaky, tender flesh. With its refreshing and herbaceous notes, the dill sauce adds a delightful burst of flavor to every bite. This dish is a visual feast and a celebration of simplicity and sophistication on your plate.

Ingredients:

For the Pan-Seared Salmon:

• Four salmon fillets, skin-on

• Salt and black pepper to taste

• Two tablespoons of olive oil

• One lemon, sliced for garnish

For the Dill Sauce:

• 1/2 cup plain Greek yogurt

• Two tablespoons fresh dill, finely chopped

• One tablespoon Dijon mustard

- One tablespoon of lemon juice

- One clove of garlic, minced

- Salt and black pepper to taste

Instructions:

Prepare the Dill Sauce:

Whisk together Greek yogurt, chopped fresh dill, Dijon mustard, lemon juice, minced garlic, salt, and black pepper in a small bowl.

Refrigerate the sauce while preparing and cooking the salmon to allow the flavors to meld.

Pan-Seared Salmon:

Pat the salmon fillets dry with paper towels. Season both sides with salt and black pepper.

Heat olive oil over medium-high heat in a large skillet until shimmering but not smoking.

Place the salmon fillets in the skillet, skin-side down. Cook for 4-5 minutes until the skin is crispy and golden.

Carefully flip the fillets and cook for an additional 3-4 minutes or until the salmon reaches your desired level of doneness. The internal temperature should be 145°F (63°C).

Remove the salmon from the skillet and let it rest for a few minutes.

Serve:

Arrange the pan-seared salmon fillets on serving plates.

Drizzle the prepared dill sauce over the salmon.

Garnish with lemon slices for an extra burst of freshness.

Serve immediately, and enjoy this elegant and flavorful pan-seared salmon with dill sauce!

Nutrition Information (per serving): Calories: 320 Protein: 35g Carbohydrates: 3g Fat: 18g Saturated Fat: 3g Cholesterol: 90mg Sodium: 220mg Fiber: 1g Sugar: 1g

STIR-FRIED BEEF WITH BROCCOLI AND SNOW PEAS

Meal Description: Indulge in the savory goodness of this quick and delicious stir-fried beef dish featuring crisp broccoli and tender snow peas. The thinly sliced beef is seared to perfection, and the vibrant vegetables are tossed in a flavorful stir-fry sauce, creating a wholesome and satisfying meal that's perfect for busy weeknights.

Ingredients:

For the Stir-Fry:

• 1 pound (450g) flank steak, thinly sliced

• 2 cups broccoli florets

• 1 cup snow peas, ends trimmed

• Three tablespoons vegetable oil, divided

• Three cloves garlic, minced

• One tablespoon of fresh ginger, grated

• Sesame seeds and sliced green onions for garnish (optional)

For the Stir-Fry Sauce:

• 1/4 cup low-sodium soy sauce

- Two tablespoons of oyster sauce

- One tablespoon of hoisin sauce

- One tablespoon of rice vinegar

- One tablespoon cornstarch

- One teaspoon of brown sugar

- 1/2 cup beef broth or water

Instructions:

Prepare the Stir-Fry Sauce:

Whisk together soy sauce, oyster sauce, hoisin sauce, rice vinegar, cornstarch, brown sugar, and beef broth in a bowl. Set aside.

Stir-Fry the Beef:

Heat 2 tablespoons of vegetable oil in a wok or large skillet over high heat.

Add the thinly sliced beef to the hot pan, spreading it out to ensure even cooking. Stir-fry for 2-3 minutes or until the meat is browned and cooked to your liking. Remove the meat from the pan and set aside.

Cook the Vegetables:

In the same pan, add the remaining one tablespoon of oil.

Stir in minced garlic and grated ginger. Cook for about 30 seconds until aromatic.

Add broccoli florets and snow peas to the pan. Stir-fry for 3-4 minutes until the vegetables are tender-crisp.

Combine and Finish:

Return the cooked beef to the pan with the vegetables.

Pour the prepared stir-fry sauce over the beef and vegetables. Toss everything together until well-coated and heated through.

If desired, garnish with sesame seeds and sliced green onions.

Serve:

Serve the stir-fried beef with broccoli and snow peas over steamed rice or noodles.

Enjoy this flavorful and nutritious stir-fry that's sure to become a favorite!

Nutrition Information (per serving, without rice or noodles): Calories: 350 Protein: 30g Carbohydrates: 14g Fat: 20g Saturated Fat: 5g Cholesterol: 70mg Sodium: 800mg Fiber: 4g Sugar: 5g

LEMON GARLIC SHRIMP SKEWERS

Meal Description: Elevate your seafood experience with these succulent Lemon Garlic Shrimp Skewers. Jumbo shrimp are marinated in a zesty blend of lemon, garlic, and herbs, then threaded onto skewers and grilled to perfection. The result is a dish bursting with bright flavors, perfect for a light and refreshing meal.

Ingredients:

For the Lemon Garlic Marinade:

- 1/4 cup olive oil

- Three tablespoons fresh lemon juice

- Two cloves garlic, minced

- One teaspoon of lemon zest

- One teaspoon dried oregano

- One teaspoon of dried parsley

- Salt and black pepper to taste

For the Shrimp Skewers:

- 1 pound (450g) jumbo shrimp, peeled and deveined

- Wooden or metal skewers (if using wooden skewers, soak them in water for 30 minutes before grilling)

For Garnish:

• Fresh parsley, chopped

• Lemon wedges

Instructions:

Prepare the Lemon Garlic Marinade:

Whisk together olive oil, fresh lemon juice, minced garlic, lemon zest, dried oregano, parsley, salt, and black pepper in a bowl.

Marinate the Shrimp:

Place the peeled and deveined shrimp in a resealable plastic bag or shallow dish.

Pour the lemon garlic marinade over the shrimp, ensuring they are well-coated. Marinate in the refrigerator for at least 15-30 minutes.

Skewer the Shrimp:

Preheat the grill to medium-high heat.

Thread the marinated shrimp onto skewers, ensuring they are evenly spaced.

Grill the Shrimp:

Place the shrimp skewers on the preheated grill.

Grill for 2-3 minutes per side or until the shrimp are opaque and lightly charred.

Garnish and Serve:

Remove the shrimp skewers from the grill.

Sprinkle with freshly chopped parsley and serve with lemon wedges on the side.

Serve:

Arrange the Lemon Garlic Shrimp Skewers on a platter.

Serve immediately, and enjoy these delightful skewers as a main dish, appetizer, or over a bed of rice or salad.

Nutrition Information (per serving): Calories: 180 Protein: 25g Carbohydrates: 2g Fat: 8g Saturated Fat: 1g Cholesterol: 180mg Sodium: 280mg Fiber: 0g Sugar: 0g

HERB-MARINATED GRILLED LAMB CHOPS

Meal Description: Savor the robust flavors of these Herb-Marinated Grilled Lamb Chops, where succulent lamb chops are infused with a medley of aromatic herbs and grilled to perfection. This dish is a celebration of simplicity and sophistication, showcasing the natural richness of lamb enhanced by a flavorful herb marinade. Ideal for a special occasion or a gourmet dinner at home.

Ingredients:

For the Herb Marinade:

- 1/4 cup olive oil

- Three tablespoons fresh rosemary, chopped

- Two tablespoons fresh thyme, chopped

- Four cloves garlic, minced

- Zest of 1 lemon

- Salt and black pepper to taste

For the Lamb Chops:

- Eight lamb chops, frenched

- Salt and black pepper to taste

For Garnish:

• Fresh mint leaves, chopped

• Lemon wedges

Instructions:

Prepare the Herb Marinade:

In a bowl, combine olive oil, chopped rosemary, chopped thyme, minced garlic, lemon zest, salt, and black pepper. Mix well to create the herb marinade.

Marinate the Lamb Chops:

Pat the lamb chops dry with paper towels. Season them with salt and black pepper on both sides.

Place the lamb chops in a shallow dish or resealable plastic bag.

Pour the herb marinade over the lamb chops, ensuring they are well-coated. Marinate in the refrigerator for at least 2 hours, allowing the flavors to meld.

Preheat the Grill:

Preheat your grill to medium-high heat.

Grill the Lamb Chops:

Remove the lamb chops from the marinade and let any excess drip off.

Grill the lamb chops for 3-4 minutes per side for medium-rare, or adjust the cooking time based on your preferred level of doneness.

Allow the lamb chops to rest for a few minutes before serving.

Garnish and Serve:

Sprinkle chopped fresh mint over the grilled lamb chops.

Serve with lemon wedges on the side.

Serve:

Arrange the Herb-Marinated Grilled Lamb Chops on a platter.

Serve immediately, and enjoy this gourmet dish with its aromatic herb infusion and perfectly grilled lamb.

Nutrition Information (per serving): Calories: 280 Protein: 25g Carbohydrates: 1g Fat: 19g Saturated Fat: 6g Cholesterol: 90mg Sodium: 80mg Fiber: 0g Sugar: 0g

TURKEY AND VEGETABLE STIR-FRY

Meal Description: Enjoy a wholesome and colorful Turkey and Vegetable Stir-Fry, where lean ground turkey is stir-fried with a vibrant array of vegetables, creating a delicious and nutritious meal. This quick and easy stir-fry is packed with protein, fiber, and a medley of flavors. Serve it over rice or noodles for a satisfying and well-balanced dish.

Ingredients:

For the Stir-Fry:

• 1 pound (450g) lean ground turkey

• Two tablespoons of vegetable oil

• One onion, thinly sliced

• Two bell peppers (different colors), sliced

• 1 cup broccoli florets

• 1 cup snap peas, trimmed

• Three cloves garlic, minced

• One tablespoon of fresh ginger, grated

• Salt and black pepper to taste

• Sesame seeds and sliced green onions for garnish (optional)

For the Stir-Fry Sauce:

• Three tablespoons of low-sodium soy sauce

• Two tablespoons of oyster sauce

• One tablespoon of hoisin sauce

• One tablespoon of rice vinegar

• One tablespoon cornstarch

• One teaspoon of brown sugar

• 1/2 cup chicken broth

Instructions:

Prepare the Stir-Fry Sauce:

Whisk together soy sauce, oyster sauce, hoisin sauce, rice vinegar, cornstarch, brown sugar, and chicken broth in a bowl. Set aside.

Stir-Fry the Turkey:

In a wok or large skillet, heat vegetable oil over medium-high heat.

Add ground turkey to the hot pan, breaking it apart with a spatula. Cook until browned and cooked through.

Remove any excess liquid released by the turkey.

Cook the Vegetables:

Add sliced onions, bell peppers, broccoli florets, and snap peas to the pan. Stir-fry for 4-5 minutes until the vegetables are crisp-tender.

Add minced garlic and grated ginger to the pan.

Cook for an additional 1-2 minutes until aromatic.

Combine and Finish:

Pour the prepared stir-fry sauce over the turkey and vegetables. Toss everything together until well-coated and heated through.

Season with salt and black pepper to taste.

Garnish and Serve:

Garnish the Turkey and Vegetable Stir-Fry with sesame seeds and sliced green onions if desired.

Serve over steamed rice or noodles.

Serve:

Dish out this flavorful and nutritious Turkey and Vegetable Stir-Fry onto plates or bowls.

Enjoy this quick and delicious stir-fry that's perfect for a wholesome weeknight dinner!

Nutrition Information (per serving, without rice or noodles): Calories: 280 Protein: 30g Carbohydrates: 15g Fat: 12g Saturated Fat: 2g Cholesterol: 60mg Sodium: 800mg Fiber: 4g Sugar: 6g

OVEN-BAKED COD WITH HERBED QUINOA

Meal Description: Experience a delightful fusion of flavors and textures with this Oven-Baked Cod served over a bed of Herbed Quinoa. The cod is seasoned with aromatic herbs, baked to perfection, and paired with a light and fluffy quinoa infused with fresh herbs. This wholesome dish is nutritious and a celebration of simplicity and sophistication on your plate.

Ingredients:

For the Baked Cod:

- Four cod fillets
- Two tablespoons of olive oil
- One tablespoon of fresh lemon juice
- One teaspoon of dried thyme
- One teaspoon of dried rosemary
- One teaspoon paprika
- Salt and black pepper to taste
- Lemon wedges for serving

For the Herbed Quinoa:

- 1 cup quinoa, rinsed and drained
- 2 cups vegetable broth or water
- Two tablespoons fresh parsley, chopped
- One tablespoon of fresh dill, chopped
- One tablespoon of fresh chives chopped
- Salt and black pepper to taste

For Garnish:

- Fresh parsley, chopped

Instructions:

Prepare the Baked Cod:

Preheat the oven to 400°F (200°C).

Mix olive oil, lemon juice, dried thyme, rosemary, paprika, salt, and black pepper in a small bowl to create the marinade.

Place the cod fillets in a baking dish. Brush each fillet with the herb-infused marinade, ensuring they are well-coated.

Bake in the preheated oven for 12-15 minutes or until the cod is opaque and flakes easily with a fork.

Prepare the Herbed Quinoa:

In a saucepan, combine quinoa and vegetable broth or water. Bring to a boil, then reduce heat to low, cover, and simmer for 15-20 minutes or until the quinoa is cooked and liquid is absorbed.

Fluff the quinoa with a fork and stir in chopped parsley, dill, chives, salt, and black pepper.

Serve:

> Arrange a portion of herbed quinoa on each plate.
>
> Place a baked cod fillet on top of the quinoa.
>
> Garnish with additional chopped fresh parsley.
>
> Serve with lemon wedges on the side.

Enjoy:

> Indulge in this Oven-Baked Cod with Herbed Quinoa, a delightful and nutritious meal that's both comforting and elegant.

Nutrition Information (per serving): Calories: 320 Protein: 30g Carbohydrates: 25g Fat: 12g Saturated Fat: 2g Cholesterol: 60mg Sodium: 600mg Fiber: 4g Sugar: 1g

CHAPTER THREE

Beneficial Grains Recipes

Quinoa Salad with Roasted Vegetables

Meal Description: Delight in this Quinoa Salad's vibrant flavors and wholesome goodness with Roasted Vegetables. Nutrient-packed quinoa is paired with a colorful medley of roasted vegetables, creating a satisfying dish that's perfect for lunch or a light dinner. The combination of textures and flavors and a zesty dressing make this salad a delightful and nutritious choice.

Ingredients:

For the Quinoa Salad:

• 1 cup quinoa, rinsed and drained

• 2 cups water or vegetable broth

• One medium zucchini, diced

• One red bell pepper, diced

• One yellow bell pepper, diced

• 1 cup cherry tomatoes, halved

• One red onion, thinly sliced

• Two tablespoons of olive oil

• Salt and black pepper to taste

• 1/4 cup fresh parsley, chopped

• 1/4 cup feta cheese, crumbled (optional)

For the Dressing:

• Three tablespoons olive oil

• Two tablespoons of balsamic vinegar

- One clove of garlic, minced

- One teaspoon of Dijon mustard

- Salt and black pepper to taste

Instructions:

Roast the Vegetables:

Preheat the oven to 400°F (200°C).

Toss diced zucchini, red bell pepper, yellow bell pepper, cherry tomatoes, and sliced red onion with olive oil, salt, and black pepper in a large bowl.

Spread the vegetables on a baking sheet in a single layer.

Roast in the preheated oven for 20-25 minutes or until the vegetables are tender and slightly caramelized. Stir occasionally for even roasting.

Prepare the Quinoa:

In a saucepan, combine quinoa and water or vegetable broth. Bring to a boil, then reduce heat to low, cover, and simmer for 15-20 minutes or until the quinoa is cooked and liquid is absorbed.

Fluff the quinoa with a fork and let it cool to room temperature.

Make the Dressing:

Whisk together olive oil, balsamic vinegar, minced garlic, Dijon mustard, salt, and black pepper in a small bowl.

Assemble the Quinoa Salad:

Combine the cooked quinoa, roasted vegetables, and chopped fresh parsley in a large serving bowl.

Drizzle the dressing over the salad and toss gently to coat all ingredients.

Garnish and Serve:

If desired, sprinkle crumbled feta cheese over the top.

Serve the Quinoa Salad with Roasted Vegetables at room temperature or chilled.

Enjoy:

Relish in the delightful flavors and textures of this nutritious and colorful quinoa salad!

Nutrition Information (per serving): Calories: 280 Protein: 8g Carbohydrates: 35g Fat: 12g Saturated Fat: 2g Cholesterol: 5mg Sodium: 250mg Fiber: 6g Sugar: 4g

BROWN RICE AND BLACK BEAN BURRITO BOWL

Meal Description: This Brown Rice and Black Bean Burrito Bowl satisfies your craving for a wholesome and flavorful meal. Packed with fiber, protein, and vibrant colors, this bowl combines nutty brown rice, seasoned black beans, and a variety of fresh toppings. Customize it to your liking with avocado, salsa, and a zesty lime-cilantro dressing for a delicious and nutritious feast.

Ingredients:

For the Brown Rice and Black Beans:

• 1 cup brown rice

• 2 cups water

• One can (15 ounces) black beans, drained and rinsed

• One teaspoon of ground cumin

• One teaspoon of chili powder

• Salt to taste

For the Burrito Bowl Toppings:

• 1 cup corn kernels (fresh, frozen, or canned)

• 1 cup cherry tomatoes, halved

- One ripe avocado, sliced

- 1 cup shredded lettuce or cabbage

- 1/2 cup red onion, finely diced

For the Lime-Cilantro Dressing:

- Three tablespoons olive oil

- Juice of 2 limes

- Two tablespoons fresh cilantro, chopped

- One teaspoon of honey or agave syrup

- Salt and black pepper to taste

Instructions:

Cook the Brown Rice:

In a saucepan, combine brown rice and water. Bring to a boil, then reduce heat to low, cover, and simmer for 40-45 minutes or until the rice is tender and water is absorbed.

Fluff the brown rice with a fork and set aside.

Prepare the Black Beans:

Combine black beans, ground cumin, chili powder, and salt in a small saucepan. Heat over medium-low until the beans are heated, and the spices are well incorporated.

Make the Lime-Cilantro Dressing:

Whisk together olive oil, lime juice, chopped cilantro, honey or agave syrup, salt, and black pepper in a small bowl. Set aside.

Assemble the Burrito Bowl:

In serving bowls, layer the cooked brown rice and

seasoned black beans.

Arrange corn kernels, cherry tomatoes, avocado slices, shredded lettuce or cabbage, and diced red onion on top.

Drizzle with Dressing:

Drizzle the lime-cilantro dressing over the burrito bowl.

Garnish and Serve:

Garnish with additional cilantro and lime wedges if desired.

Serve immediately and enjoy this flavorful and nutritious Brown Rice and Black Bean Burrito Bowl!

Nutrition Information (per serving): Calories: 450 Protein: 12g Carbohydrates: 70g Fat: 15g Saturated Fat: 2g Cholesterol: 0mg Sodium: 300mg Fiber: 12g Sugar: 5g

MILLET PILAF WITH SPINACH AND PINE NUTS

Meal Description: Elevate your grain game with this Millet Pilaf featuring vibrant spinach and toasty pine nuts. This wholesome dish is a symphony of flavors and textures, with nutty millet, tender spinach, and crunchy pine nuts coming together in a delightful medley. Serve as a side dish or a light main course for a nutritious and satisfying meal.

Ingredients:

For the Millet Pilaf:

• 1 cup millet, rinsed and drained

• 2 cups vegetable broth or water

• One tablespoon of olive oil

• One small onion, finely chopped

• Two cloves garlic, minced

• 1 cup fresh spinach, chopped

• 1/4 cup pine nuts, toasted

• Salt and black pepper to taste

For Garnish:

- Fresh parsley, chopped

- Lemon wedges

Instructions:

Cook the Millet:

In a saucepan, combine millet and vegetable broth or water. Bring to a boil, then reduce heat to low, cover, and simmer for 15-20 minutes or until the millet is cooked and liquid is absorbed.

Fluff the millet with a fork and let it cool slightly.

Toast the Pine Nuts:

In a dry skillet over medium heat, toast the pine nuts until golden brown and fragrant. Be attentive, as they can quickly go from toasted to burnt.

Prepare the Millet Pilaf:

In a large skillet, heat olive oil over medium heat.

Add chopped onion and sauté until softened and translucent.

Stir in minced garlic and cook for an additional 1-2 minutes until aromatic.

Add the cooked millet to the skillet, tossing to combine with the onion and garlic.

Fold in chopped spinach and toasted pine nuts. Cook for 2-3 minutes until the spinach is wilted.

Season with salt and black pepper to taste.

Garnish and Serve:

Garnish the Millet Pilaf with chopped fresh parsley.

Serve with lemon wedges on the side for a burst of citrus flavor.

Enjoy:

Enjoy this Millet Pilaf with Spinach and Pine Nuts as a nutritious side dish or a light main course.

Serve warm and savor the delightful combination of nutty millet, earthy spinach, and the crunch of toasted pine nuts.

Nutrition Information (per serving): Calories: 280 Protein: 8g Carbohydrates: 40g Fat: 10g Saturated Fat: 1g Cholesterol: 0mg Sodium: 400mg Fiber: 5g Sugar: 1g

BUCKWHEAT STIR-FRY WITH TOFU AND VEGETABLES

Meal Description: Embark on a flavorful journey with this Buckwheat Stir-Fry featuring protein-packed tofu and a colorful array of vegetables. Buckwheat, rich in nutrients, forms the base of this wholesome dish. Tossed with savory stir-fried tofu and an assortment of crisp vegetables, this stir-fry is both nutritious and satisfying. Enjoy the unique nutty taste of buckwheat in every bite!

Ingredients:

For the Buckwheat Stir-Fry:

• 1 cup buckwheat groats, rinsed and drained

• 2 cups vegetable broth

• One tablespoon of sesame oil

• One block (14 ounces) of extra-firm tofu, pressed and cubed

• 1 cup broccoli florets

• One bell pepper, thinly sliced (any color)

• One carrot, julienned

• Two cloves garlic, minced

- One tablespoon ginger, grated
- 1/4 cup soy sauce or tamari
- One tablespoon of rice vinegar
- One tablespoon of maple syrup or agave syrup
- Two green onions, sliced
- Sesame seeds for garnish

Instructions:

Cook the Buckwheat:

In a saucepan, bring vegetable broth to a boil.

Add rinsed buckwheat groats, reduce heat to low, cover, and simmer for 15-20 minutes or until buckwheat is tender and liquid is absorbed.

Fluff the buckwheat with a fork and set aside.

Prepare the Tofu:

In a large skillet or wok, heat sesame oil over medium-high heat.

Add cubed tofu and stir-fry until golden brown on all sides. Remove tofu from the skillet and set aside.

Stir-Fry the Vegetables:

Add broccoli, bell pepper, and julienned carrot in the same skillet. Stir-fry for 3-4 minutes until the vegetables are crisp-tender.

Add minced garlic and grated ginger to the vegetables. Cook for an additional 1-2 minutes until aromatic.

Combine and Sauce:

Return the cooked buckwheat and stir-fried tofu to the skillet with the vegetables.

Mix soy sauce, rice vinegar, and maple syrup in a small bowl. Pour the sauce over the buckwheat, tofu, and vegetables.

Toss everything together until well-coated and heated through.

Garnish and Serve:

Garnish the Buckwheat Stir-Fry with sliced green onions and sesame seeds.

Serve immediately and enjoy the nutty goodness of this nutritious and flavorful stir-fry!

Nutrition Information (per serving): Calories: 350 Protein: 15g Carbohydrates: 55g Fat: 8g Saturated Fat: 1g Cholesterol: 0mg Sodium: 800mg Fiber: 8g Sugar: 6g

WILD RICE AND MUSHROOM STUFFED BELL PEPPERS

Meal Description: Delight your taste buds with these Wild Rice and Mushroom Stuffed Bell Peppers, a wholesome and flavorful dish that brings together the nutty goodness of wild rice and the earthy richness of mushrooms. These stuffed peppers are a visual feast and a nutritious and satisfying meal that captures the essence of comfort food with a healthy twist.

Ingredients:

For the Stuffed Bell Peppers:

• Four large bell peppers, halved and seeds removed

• 1 cup wild rice, cooked according to package instructions

• One tablespoon of olive oil

• One onion, finely chopped

• Two cloves garlic, minced

• 8 ounces (about 225g) mushrooms, finely chopped

- One teaspoon of dried thyme

- One teaspoon dried oregano

- Salt and black pepper to taste

- 1/4 cup fresh parsley, chopped

- 1/2 cup grated Parmesan cheese (optional)

For Garnish:

- Fresh parsley, chopped

Instructions:

Preheat the Oven:

Preheat the oven to 375°F (190°C).

Prepare the Bell Peppers:

Cut the bell peppers in half lengthwise, removing the seeds and membranes. Place them in a baking dish.

Cook the Wild Rice:

Cook the wild rice according to package instructions. Set aside.

Saute the Vegetables:

In a large skillet, heat olive oil over medium heat.

Add finely chopped onion and sauté until softened and translucent.

Stir in minced garlic and cook for an additional 1-2 minutes until aromatic.

Add chopped mushrooms to the skillet and cook until they release their moisture and become tender.

Combine the Filling:

Combine the cooked wild rice with the sautéed mushroom mixture in a bowl.

Add dried thyme, dried oregano, salt, black pepper, and chopped fresh parsley. Mix well.

Optionally, mix in grated Parmesan cheese for added richness.

Stuff the Bell Peppers:

Generously stuff each bell pepper half with the wild rice and mushroom mixture.

Press the filling down slightly and mound it on top.

Bake:

Cover the baking dish with foil and bake in the preheated oven for 25-30 minutes or until the peppers are tender.

Uncover and bake for an additional 5-10 minutes for a golden top.

Garnish and Serve:

Garnish the Wild Rice and Mushroom Stuffed Bell Peppers with chopped fresh parsley.

Serve warm and enjoy this wholesome and flavorful stuffed peppers dish!

Nutrition Information (per serving): Calories: 250 Protein: 7g Carbohydrates: 45g Fat: 6g Saturated Fat: 1g Cholesterol: 5mg Sodium: 300mg Fiber: 6g Sugar: 6g

AMARANTH BREAKFAST PORRIDGE WITH BERRIES

Meal Description: Start your day with a nutritious and delightful Amaranth Breakfast Porridge featuring the earthy goodness of Amaranth grains and the vibrant sweetness of mixed berries. This wholesome porridge is a hearty and satisfying breakfast option that provides a burst of energy, fiber, and antioxidants. It's not only nourishing but also a feast for the senses.

Ingredients:

For the Amaranth Porridge:

- 1/2 cup amaranth grains

- 2 cups milk (dairy or plant-based)

- One tablespoon of maple syrup or honey

- 1/2 teaspoon vanilla extract

- 1/4 teaspoon ground cinnamon

- Pinch of salt

For Topping:

- Mixed berries (strawberries, blueberries, raspberries)

- Chopped nuts (almonds, walnuts, or pistachios)

- Drizzle of honey or maple syrup

Instructions:

Rinse and Cook Amaranth:

Rinse the amaranth grains under cold water.

Combine the rinsed amaranth, milk, maple syrup or honey, vanilla extract, ground cinnamon, and a pinch of salt in a saucepan.

Bring the mixture to a boil, then reduce the heat to low, cover, and simmer for 20-25 minutes or until the amaranth is cooked and has a creamy consistency.

Prepare the Berries:

While the amaranth is cooking, wash and prepare the mixed berries.

If using strawberries, hull and slice them. Keep other berries whole or halved as needed.

Assemble the Breakfast Bowl:

Once the amaranth porridge is ready, spoon it into serving bowls.

Top the porridge with a generous amount of mixed berries.

Add Nutty Crunch:

Sprinkle chopped nuts (almonds, walnuts, or pistachios) over the berries for a nutty crunch.

Drizzle with Sweetness:

Drizzle a bit of honey or maple syrup over the top for added sweetness.

Serve and Enjoy:

Serve the Amaranth Breakfast Porridge with Berries immediately while warm.

Enjoy this nourishing and flavorful breakfast that combines the wholesome goodness of amaranth with the freshness of mixed berries!

Nutrition Information (per serving): Calories: 300 Protein: 8g Carbohydrates: 50g Fat: 8g Saturated Fat: 2g Cholesterol: 10mg Sodium: 120mg Fiber: 7g Sugar: 15g

SORGHUM AND CHICKPEA SALAD WITH LEMON VINAIGRETTE

Meal Description: Delight in the wholesome goodness of this Sorghum and Chickpea Salad, a refreshing and protein-packed dish featuring nutty sorghum grains and hearty chickpeas. Tossed with a zesty lemon vinaigrette, this salad is a burst of flavors and textures, offering a nutritious and satisfying meal that's perfect for lunch or as a vibrant side dish.

Ingredients:

For the Sorghum and Chickpea Salad:

• 1 cup sorghum grains, cooked according to package instructions

• One can (15 ounces) chickpeas, drained and rinsed

• One cucumber, diced

• One red bell pepper, diced

• 1/2 red onion, finely chopped

• 1/4 cup fresh parsley, chopped

• 1/4 cup feta cheese, crumbled (optional)

• Salt and black pepper to taste

For the Lemon Vinaigrette:

• 1/4 cup olive oil

• Juice of 2 lemons

• One teaspoon of Dijon mustard

• One clove of garlic, minced

• 1 teaspoon honey or agave syrup

• Salt and black pepper to taste

Instructions:

Cook Sorghum:

Cook sorghum grains according to package instructions. Once cooked, let them cool to room temperature.

Prepare Chickpeas:

In a colander, rinse canned chickpeas under cold water. Drain well.

Assemble the Salad:

Combine cooked sorghum, chickpeas, diced cucumber, red bell pepper, chopped red onion, and chopped fresh parsley in a large bowl.

If using, sprinkle crumbled feta cheese over the salad.

Season with salt and black pepper to taste.

Make Lemon Vinaigrette:

Whisk together olive oil, lemon juice, Dijon mustard, minced garlic, honey or agave syrup, salt, and black pepper in a small bowl.

Dress the Salad:

Pour the lemon vinaigrette over the sorghum and chickpea salad.

Toss everything together until well-coated with the vinaigrette.

Chill and Serve:

Refrigerate the salad for at least 30 minutes to allow the flavors to meld.

Serve chilled, and enjoy the Sorghum and Chickpea Salad as a nutritious and flavorful meal.

Nutrition Information (per serving): Calories: 320 Protein: 10g Carbohydrates: 45g Fat: 12g Saturated Fat: 2g Cholesterol: 5mg Sodium: 300mg Fiber: 8g Sugar: 4g

TEFF PANCAKES WITH BLUEBERRY COMPOTE

Meal Description: Indulge in a wholesome and delicious breakfast with Teff pancakes topped with a luscious blueberry soup. Teff, a nutrient-rich ancient grain, lends these pancakes a unique nutty flavor and hearty texture. Paired with the vibrant sweetness of the blueberry compote, this breakfast treat is satisfying and a delightful way to start your day.

Ingredients:

For the Teff Pancakes:

- 1 cup teff flour

- One tablespoon sugar

- One teaspoon of baking powder

- 1/2 teaspoon baking soda

- 1/4 teaspoon salt

- 1 cup buttermilk

- One large egg

- Two tablespoons melted butter or oil

- One teaspoon of vanilla extract

For the Blueberry Compote:

- 1 cup blueberries (fresh or frozen)
- Two tablespoons of maple syrup or honey
- One tablespoon water
- One teaspoon of lemon juice
- Zest of half a lemon

Instructions:

Prepare the Teff Pancake Batter:

Whisk together teff flour, sugar, baking powder, baking soda, and salt in a large bowl.

Whisk together buttermilk, egg, melted butter or oil, and vanilla extract in a separate bowl.

Pour the wet ingredients into the dry ingredients and stir until just combined. Let the batter rest for a few minutes.

Cook the Teff Pancakes:

Heat a griddle or non-stick skillet over medium heat. Lightly grease with cooking spray or butter.

Pour 1/4 cup portions of batter onto the griddle for each pancake. Cook until bubbles form on the surface, then flip and cook until golden brown on the other side.

Repeat until all the batter is used, keeping the cooked pancakes warm.

Make the Blueberry Compote:

Combine blueberries, maple syrup or honey, water, lemon juice, and lemon zest in a small saucepan.

Cook over medium heat, stirring occasionally, until the blueberries burst and the mixture thickens into a compote. This will take about 5-7 minutes.

Remove from heat and let it cool slightly.

Serve:

Stack the Teff Pancakes on a plate and generously spoon the warm Blueberry Compote over the top.

Optionally, drizzle with additional maple syrup or honey.

Enjoy:

Indulge in the delightful combination of Teff Pancakes and Blueberry Compote for a satisfying and flavorful breakfast!

Nutrition Information (per serving, without additional toppings): Calories: 250 Protein: 6g Carbohydrates: 40g Fat: 8g Saturated Fat: 4g Cholesterol: 50mg Sodium: 400mg Fiber: 5g Sugar: 15g

CHAPTER FOUR

Certain Legumes Recipes

Lentil and Kale Soup

Meal Description: Warm up your day with a nourishing bowl of Lentil and Kale Soup, a hearty and wholesome dish that combines protein-rich lentils with the nutritional powerhouse, kale. Packed with vegetables and aromatic spices, this soup provides comfort and a myriad of essential nutrients. Enjoy the robust flavors and the health benefits of this delicious homemade soup.

Ingredients:

For the Lentil and Kale Soup:

• 1 cup dried green or brown lentils, rinsed and drained

• One tablespoon of olive oil

• One onion, diced

• Two carrots diced

• Two celery stalks, diced

• Three cloves garlic, minced

• One teaspoon of ground cumin

• One teaspoon of ground coriander

• 1/2 teaspoon smoked paprika

• One bay leaf

• 6 cups vegetable broth

• One can (14 ounces) diced tomatoes

• 4 cups kale, stemmed and chopped

• Salt and black pepper to taste

• Fresh lemon wedges for serving

Instructions:

Prepare Lentils:

Rinse lentils under cold water and set aside.

Saute Aromatics:

In a large pot, heat olive oil over medium heat.

Add diced onion, carrots, and celery. Saute for 5-7 minutes until vegetables are softened.

Stir in minced garlic, ground cumin, ground coriander, smoked paprika, and bay leaf. Cook for an additional 1-2 minutes until fragrant.

Simmer Soup:

Pour vegetable broth into the pot, followed by diced tomatoes and rinsed lentils.

Bring the soup to a boil, then reduce heat to low, cover, and simmer for 25-30 minutes or until lentils are tender.

Add Kale:

Stir in chopped kale and continue to simmer for an additional 5-7 minutes until the kale is wilted and tender.

Season and Serve:

Season the soup with salt and black pepper to taste.

Remove the bay leaf before serving.

Serve with Lemon:

Ladle the Lentil and Kale Soup into bowls.

Serve with fresh lemon wedges on the side for a citrusy touch.

Enjoy:

Enjoy this nourishing Lentil and Kale Soup as a comforting meal, providing a perfect balance of protein, fiber, and essential vitamins!

Nutrition Information (per serving): Calories: 250 Protein: 15g Carbohydrates: 45g Fat: 3g Saturated Fat: 0.5g Cholesterol: 0mg Sodium: 800mg Fiber: 12g Sugar: 6g

ADZUKI BEAN AND VEGETABLE STIR-FRY

Meal Description: Savor the flavors of this nutritious and vibrant Adzuki Bean and Vegetable Stir-Fry, where protein-packed adzuki beans meet a colorful assortment of crisp vegetables. This stir-fry is a feast for the senses and a wholesome dish that brings together the goodness of plant-based proteins and nutrient-rich veggies. Enjoy the delightful combination of textures and flavors in every bite!

Ingredients:

For the Stir-Fry:

- 1 cup adzuki beans, cooked
- Two tablespoons of sesame oil
- One onion, thinly sliced
- Two carrots julienned
- One bell pepper (any color), thinly sliced
- One zucchini, thinly sliced
- 2 cups broccoli florets
- Three cloves garlic, minced

- One tablespoon of fresh ginger, grated
- 1/4 cup soy sauce or tamari
- One tablespoon of rice vinegar
- One tablespoon of maple syrup or agave syrup
- One teaspoon of sesame seeds for garnish
- Green onions, sliced, for garnish

Instructions:

Prepare Adzuki Beans:

If using dried adzuki beans, cook them according to package instructions until they are tender. If using canned beans, rinse and drain them.

Stir-Fry Vegetables:

Heat sesame oil in a wok or large skillet over medium-high heat.

Add thinly sliced onion, julienned carrots, sliced bell pepper, sliced zucchini, and broccoli florets. Stir-fry for 5-7 minutes until the vegetables are crisp-tender.

Add minced garlic and grated ginger to the vegetables, and stir-fry for an additional 1-2 minutes until aromatic.

Add Adzuki Beans:

Toss in the cooked adzuki beans and stir to combine with the vegetables.

Prepare Sauce:

Mix soy sauce or tamari, rice vinegar, and maple syrup or agave syrup in a small bowl to create the sauce.

Pour the sauce over the stir-fry and toss everything together until well-coated.

Garnish and Serve:

Sprinkle sesame seeds and sliced green onions over the top for garnish.

Stir for an additional minute to ensure the sauce is evenly distributed.

Serve Hot:

Serve the Adzuki Bean and Vegetable Stir-Fry hot over a bed of rice or your favorite grain.

Enjoy:

Enjoy this plant-powered stir-fry as a nutritious and flavorful meal that's both satisfying and good for you!

Nutrition Information (per serving): Calories: 280 Protein: 12g Carbohydrates: 40g Fat: 10g Saturated Fat: 1.5g Cholesterol: 0mg Sodium: 800mg Fiber: 10g Sugar: 8g

BLACK-EYED PEA SALAD WITH TOMATOES AND CUCUMBERS

Meal Description: Refresh your palate with the vibrant flavors of this Black-Eyed Pea Salad, a light and nutritious dish featuring protein-packed black-eyed peas, juicy tomatoes, and crisp cucumbers. Dressed in a zesty vinaigrette, this salad is a feast for the eyes and a delightful combination of textures and tastes. Enjoy the freshness of this wholesome salad as a side dish or a light main course.

Ingredients:

For the Black-Eyed Pea Salad:

• 2 cups cooked black-eyed peas (canned or freshly cooked)

• 1 cup cherry tomatoes, halved

• One cucumber, diced

• 1/2 red onion, finely chopped

• 1/4 cup fresh parsley, chopped

- 1/4 cup fresh mint, chopped (optional)

- 1/2 cup feta cheese, crumbled (optional)

- Salt and black pepper to taste

For the Vinaigrette:

- Three tablespoons olive oil

- Two tablespoons of red wine vinegar

- One teaspoon of Dijon mustard

- One clove of garlic, minced

- One teaspoon of honey or agave syrup

- Salt and black pepper to taste

Instructions:

Prepare Black-Eyed Peas:

If using canned black-eyed peas, rinse and drain them. If using dried peas, cook according to package instructions until tender.

Assemble the Salad:

Combine the cooked black-eyed peas, cherry tomatoes, diced cucumber, finely chopped red onion, fresh parsley, and optional fresh mint in a large bowl.

If desired, sprinkle crumbled feta cheese over the top.

Season with salt and black pepper to taste.

Make the Vinaigrette:

Whisk together olive oil, red wine vinegar, Dijon mustard, minced garlic, honey or agave syrup, salt, and black pepper in a small bowl.

Dress the Salad:

Pour the vinaigrette over the black-eyed pea salad.

Toss everything together until well-coated with the vinaigrette.

Chill and Serve:

Refrigerate the salad for at least 30 minutes to allow the flavors to meld.

Serve chilled, and enjoy the Black-Eyed Pea Salad as a refreshing and nutritious addition to your meal.

Nutrition Information (per serving): Calories: 250 Protein: 9g Carbohydrates: 30g Fat: 12g Saturated Fat: 3g Cholesterol: 10mg Sodium: 300mg Fiber: 8g Sugar: 5g

RED LENTIL DAHL WITH COCONUT MILK

Meal Description: Experience the rich and comforting flavors of Red Lentil Dahl with Coconut Milk, a classic dish that combines the heartiness of red lentils with the creamy goodness of coconut milk. Infused with aromatic spices, this dahl is a perfect balance of protein, fiber, and enticing spices. Serve it over rice or with warm naan for a satisfying and nourishing meal.

Ingredients:

For the Red Lentil Dahl:

- 1 cup red lentils, rinsed and drained

- One can (14 ounces) coconut milk

- One onion, finely chopped

- Three cloves garlic, minced

- One tablespoon of fresh ginger, grated

- One can (14 ounces) diced tomatoes

- One teaspoon of ground turmeric

- One teaspoon of ground cumin

- One teaspoon of ground coriander

- 1/2 teaspoon chili powder (adjust to taste)
- One teaspoon of garam masala
- One tablespoon of vegetable oil
- Salt and black pepper to taste
- Fresh cilantro for garnish

For Serving:

- Cooked basmati rice or naan bread

Instructions:

Rinse Lentils:

Rinse red lentils under cold water until the water runs clear. Set aside.

Saute Aromatics:

In a large pot, heat vegetable oil over medium heat.

Add finely chopped onion and sauté until softened and translucent.

Stir in minced garlic and grated ginger, cooking for an additional 1-2 minutes until aromatic.

Add Spices:

Add the turmeric, cumin, coriander, chili powder, and garam masala to the pot. Stir well to coat the aromatics with the spices.

Cook Lentils:

Add rinsed red lentils to the pot, followed by coconut milk and diced tomatoes.

Season with salt and black pepper to taste.

Bring the mixture to a boil, then reduce heat to low, cover, and simmer for 20-25 minutes or until the lentils are tender and the flavors meld.

Adjust Consistency:

If the dahl is too thick, you can add a bit of water or vegetable broth to achieve your desired consistency.

Garnish and Serve:

Garnish the Red Lentil Dahl with fresh cilantro.

Serve the dahl over cooked basmati rice or with warm naan bread.

Enjoy:

Enjoy this Red Lentil Dahl with Coconut Milk for a soul-warming and satisfying meal that brings together the richness of lentils and the creaminess of coconut milk.

Nutrition Information (per serving, without rice or naan): Calories: 300 Protein: 15g Carbohydrates: 35g Fat: 14g Saturated Fat: 10g Cholesterol: 0mg Sodium: 400mg Fiber: 10g Sugar: 5g

WHITE BEAN AND ROSEMARY HUMMUS

Meal Description: Elevate your snack game with the earthy flavors of White Bean and Rosemary Hummus, a delightful twist on the classic chickpea-based dip. This hummus combines creamy white beans with the aromatic essence of fresh rosemary, creating a savory spread perfect for dipping veggie crackers or spreading on your favorite bread. Enjoy a burst of Mediterranean-inspired goodness in every bite!

Ingredients:

• One can (15 ounces) white beans (cannellini or navy), drained and rinsed

• Two cloves garlic, minced

• Two tablespoons tahini

• Three tablespoons fresh lemon juice

• One teaspoon of fresh rosemary, finely chopped

• 1/4 cup extra-virgin olive oil

• Salt and black pepper to taste

• Water (as needed for consistency)

• Optional garnish: Extra rosemary, olive oil, and a sprinkle of paprika

Instructions:

Prepare White Beans:

Drain and rinse the white beans under cold water.

Blend Ingredients:

Combine the white beans, minced garlic, tahini, fresh lemon juice, and finely chopped fresh rosemary in a food processor.

Pulse the ingredients until well combined.

Add Olive Oil:

With the food processor running, slowly drizzle in the extra-virgin olive oil. Continue to blend until the hummus reaches a smooth and creamy consistency.

Season and Adjust:

Season the hummus with salt and black pepper to taste.

If the hummus is too thick, you can add water, one tablespoon at a time, until you reach your desired consistency.

Garnish:

Transfer the hummus to a serving bowl.

Garnish with a drizzle of olive oil, a sprinkle of paprika, and additional fresh rosemary for an extra burst of flavor.

Serve:

Serve the White Bean and Rosemary Hummus

with your favorite fresh vegetables, pita bread, or crackers.

Enjoy:

Dive into the savory goodness of this Mediterranean-inspired hummus, perfect for a healthy and flavorful snack or appetizer!

Nutrition Information (per serving): Calories: 150 Protein: 5g Carbohydrates: 12g Fat: 10g Saturated Fat: 1.5g Cholesterol: 0mg Sodium: 200mg Fiber: 3g Sugar: 0g

EDAMAME AND QUINOA SALAD

Meal Description: Tantalize your taste buds with the freshness of this Edamame and Quinoa Salad, a vibrant and protein-packed dish that combines the nutty goodness of quinoa with the crunch of edamame and an array of colorful vegetables. Tossed in a zesty vinaigrette, this salad is a visual delight and a nutritious and satisfying addition to your meal. Enjoy the medley of flavors and textures in every forkful!

Ingredients:

For the Quinoa Salad:

• 1 cup quinoa, rinsed

• 2 cups water

• 1 cup edamame, shelled and cooked

• 1 cup cherry tomatoes, halved

• One cucumber, diced

• 1/2 red onion, finely chopped

• 1/4 cup fresh cilantro, chopped

• 1/4 cup feta cheese, crumbled (optional)

• Salt and black pepper to taste

For the Vinaigrette:

- Three tablespoons olive oil
- Two tablespoons of balsamic vinegar
- One teaspoon of Dijon mustard
- One clove of garlic, minced
- One teaspoon of honey or agave syrup
- Salt and black pepper to taste

Instructions:

Cook Quinoa:

In a saucepan, combine quinoa and water. Bring to a boil, then reduce heat to low, cover, and simmer for 15-20 minutes or until the quinoa is cooked and water is absorbed.

Fluff the quinoa with a fork and let it cool to room temperature.

Prepare Edamame:

Cook edamame according to package instructions. Drain and set aside.

Assemble the Salad:

Combine cooked quinoa, edamame, halved cherry tomatoes, diced cucumber, finely chopped red onion, fresh cilantro, and optional crumbled feta cheese in a large bowl.

Season with salt and black pepper to taste.

Make the Vinaigrette:

Whisk together olive oil, balsamic vinegar, Dijon mustard, minced garlic, honey or agave syrup, salt, and black pepper in a small bowl.

Dress the Salad:

Pour the vinaigrette over the quinoa salad.

Toss everything together until well-coated with the vinaigrette.

Chill and Serve:

Refrigerate the salad for at least 30 minutes to allow the flavors to meld.

Serve chilled, and enjoy the Edamame and Quinoa Salad as a wholesome and flavorful side dish or light meal.

Nutrition Information (per serving): Calories: 280 Protein: 10g Carbohydrates: 35g Fat: 12g Saturated Fat: 2g Cholesterol: 5mg Sodium: 300mg Fiber: 6g Sugar: 5g

PINTO BEAN TACOS WITH AVOCADO SALSA

Meal Description: Indulge in the savory goodness of Pinto Bean Tacos with Avocado Salsa, a plant-based delight that brings together the heartiness of seasoned pinto beans and the freshness of avocado salsa. These tacos offer a burst of flavors and textures, making them perfect for a satisfying and wholesome meal. Enjoy the combination of protein-packed beans and zesty avocado salsa in each delicious bite!

Ingredients:

For the Pinto Bean Filling:

• Two cans (15 ounces each) pinto beans, drained and rinsed

• One tablespoon of olive oil

• One onion, finely chopped

• Two cloves garlic, minced

• One teaspoon of ground cumin

• One teaspoon of smoked paprika

• 1/2 teaspoon chili powder

- Salt and black pepper to taste

- 1/4 cup water (as needed)

For the Avocado Salsa:

- Two ripe avocados, diced

- 1 cup cherry tomatoes, diced

- 1/2 red onion, finely chopped

- 1/4 cup fresh cilantro, chopped

- Juice of 1 lime

- Salt and black pepper to taste

For Assembling Tacos:

- Corn or flour tortillas

- Shredded lettuce

- Optional toppings: Shredded cheese, hot sauce, Greek yogurt or sour cream

Instructions:

Prepare Pinto Bean Filling:

In a large skillet, heat olive oil over medium heat.

Add finely chopped onion and sauté until softened.

Stir in minced garlic, ground cumin, smoked paprika, chili powder, salt, and black pepper. Cook for an additional 1-2 minutes until fragrant.

Add drained and rinsed pinto beans to the skillet. Mash some of the beans with a fork or potato masher for a chunky texture.

If the mixture is too dry, add water as needed to achieve your desired consistency. Cook for 5-7 minutes, allowing the flavors to meld.

Prepare Avocado Salsa:

Combine diced avocados, cherry tomatoes, finely chopped red onion, chopped fresh cilantro, lime juice, salt, and black pepper in a bowl. Gently toss to combine.

Assemble Tacos:

Warm the tortillas according to package instructions.

Spoon the pinto bean filling onto each tortilla.

Top with shredded lettuce and a generous scoop of avocado salsa.

Add optional toppings such as shredded cheese, hot sauce, or a dollop of Greek yogurt or sour cream.

Serve and Enjoy:

Serve the Pinto Bean Tacos with Avocado Salsa immediately, allowing everyone to customize their tacos with their favorite toppings.

Enjoy this plant-powered and flavor-packed taco feast!

Nutrition Information (per serving, without optional toppings): Calories: 300 Protein: 10g Carbohydrates: 40g Fat: 12g Saturated Fat: 2g Cholesterol: 0mg Sodium: 400mg Fiber: 12g Sugar: 2g

CHAPTER FIVE

Leafy Greens Recipes

Spinach and Feta Stuffed Chicken Breast

Meal Description: Elevate your dinner with this elegant Spinach and Feta Stuffed Chicken Breast, a delightful combination of tender chicken, sautéed spinach, and creamy feta cheese. This dish not only looks impressive but also bursts with flavors and textures. Serve it with your favorite sides for a restaurant-worthy meal that's surprisingly easy to make at home. Enjoy the savory goodness of each bite!

Ingredients:

For the Spinach and Feta Stuffing:

- 2 cups fresh spinach, chopped

- 1/2 cup feta cheese, crumbled

- Two tablespoons of olive oil

- Two cloves garlic, minced

- Salt and black pepper to taste

For the Chicken Breast:

- Four boneless, skinless chicken breasts

- One tablespoon of olive oil

- One teaspoon dried oregano

- One teaspoon of dried thyme

- Salt and black pepper to taste

- Toothpicks (to secure the stuffed chicken)

For Baking:

- One tablespoon of olive oil (for brushing)

Instructions:

Prepare Spinach and Feta Stuffing:

In a skillet, heat two tablespoons of olive oil over medium heat.

Add minced garlic and sauté until fragrant.

Add chopped spinach and cook until wilted. Season with salt and black pepper.

Remove from heat and stir in crumbled feta cheese. Set aside to cool.

Prepare Chicken Breasts:

Preheat the oven to 375°F (190°C).

Place each chicken breast between plastic wrap and pound with a meat mallet to an even thickness.

Season each chicken breast with dried oregano, dried thyme, salt, and black pepper.

Stuff Chicken Breasts:

Divide the cooled spinach and feta mixture evenly and spoon it onto the center of each chicken breast.

Carefully roll the chicken breast around the filling and secure it with toothpicks to hold the shape.

Sear and Bake:

Heat one tablespoon of olive oil over medium-high heat in an oven-safe skillet.

Sear the stuffed chicken breasts on all sides until golden brown.

Transfer the skillet to the preheated oven and bake

for 20-25 minutes or until the chicken reaches an internal temperature of 165°F (74°C).

Serve:

Remove toothpicks from the chicken before serving.

Alternatively, brush the stuffed chicken breasts with olive oil for a glossy finish.

Enjoy:

Serve the Spinach and Feta Stuffed Chicken Breast hot, and savor the delicious combination of tender chicken and flavorful filling.

Nutrition Information (per serving): Calories: 300 Protein: 35g Carbohydrates: 2g Fat: 18g Saturated Fat: 6g Cholesterol: 90mg Sodium: 400mg Fiber: 1g Sugar: 0g

KALE AND QUINOA SALAD WITH LEMON TAHINI DRESSING

Meal Description: Experience the vibrant and nutrient-packed goodness of this Kale and Quinoa Salad with Lemon Tahini Dressing. This refreshing salad combines hearty quinoa, nutrient-rich kale, and an array of colorful vegetables, all tossed in a zesty and creamy lemon tahini dressing. Packed with flavor and wholesome ingredients, this salad is a satisfying and nutritious addition to your meal. Enjoy the crispness of kale, the nuttiness of quinoa, and the tanginess of the dressing in every delightful bite!

Ingredients:

For the Salad:

- 1 cup quinoa, rinsed

- 2 cups water

- 4 cups kale, stems removed and leaves thinly sliced

- One red bell pepper, diced

- One cucumber, diced

- 1 cup cherry tomatoes, halved
- 1/2 red onion, finely chopped
- 1/4 cup fresh parsley, chopped
- 1/4 cup feta cheese, crumbled (optional)
- Salt and black pepper to taste

For the Lemon Tahini Dressing:

- 1/4 cup tahini
- Three tablespoons olive oil
- Two tablespoons of fresh lemon juice
- One clove of garlic, minced
- One teaspoon of honey or agave syrup
- Salt and black pepper to taste
- Water (as needed to thin the dressing)

Instructions:

Cook Quinoa:

In a saucepan, combine quinoa and water. Bring to a boil, then reduce heat to low, cover, and simmer for 15-20 minutes or until the quinoa is cooked and water is absorbed.

Fluff the quinoa with a fork and let it cool to room temperature.

Prepare Lemon Tahini Dressing:

Whisk together tahini, olive oil, fresh lemon juice, minced garlic, honey or agave syrup, salt, and black pepper in a bowl.

If the dressing is too thick, add water, one tablespoon at a time, until you reach your desired consistency. Set aside.

Assemble the Salad:

In a large bowl, combine cooked quinoa, sliced kale, red bell pepper, cucumber, halved cherry tomatoes, finely chopped red onion, fresh parsley, and optional crumbled feta cheese.

Season with salt and black pepper to taste.

Toss with Lemon Tahini Dressing:

Drizzle the lemon tahini dressing over the salad.

Toss everything together until well-coated with the dressing.

Chill and Serve:

Refrigerate the salad for at least 30 minutes to allow the flavors to meld.

Serve chilled, and enjoy the Kale and Quinoa Salad with Lemon Tahini Dressing as a refreshing and nutrient-rich dish.

Nutrition Information (per serving, without optional toppings): Calories: 320 Protein: 9g Carbohydrates: 35g Fat: 18g Saturated Fat: 2.5g Cholesterol: 5mg Sodium: 200mg Fiber: 6g Sugar: 3g

COLLARD GREEN WRAPS WITH TURKEY AND AVOCADO

Meal Description: Indulge in a nutritious and flavorful meal with these Collard Green Wraps featuring lean turkey, creamy avocado, and a medley of fresh vegetables. These wraps offer a satisfying crunch and a burst of colors and textures. Packed with protein, fiber, and healthy fats, these wraps are a wholesome option for a light, delicious lunch or dinner. Enjoy the goodness of nutrient-dense ingredients wrapped in vibrant collard greens!

Ingredients:

For the Collard Green Wraps:

• Four large collard green leaves stem removed

• 1 pound lean ground turkey

• One tablespoon of olive oil

• One teaspoon of ground cumin

• One teaspoon of smoked paprika

- 1/2 teaspoon garlic powder

- Salt and black pepper to taste

For the Filling:

- One avocado, sliced

- 1 cup cherry tomatoes, halved

- One cucumber, julienned

- 1/2 red onion, thinly sliced

- Fresh cilantro leaves (optional)

For the Sauce:

- 1/4 cup Greek yogurt or dairy-free alternative

- Two tablespoons of lime juice

- One tablespoon of honey or agave syrup

- Salt and black pepper to taste

Instructions:

Prepare Collard Green Leaves:

Blanch the collard green leaves in boiling water for 30 seconds to 1 minute until they become pliable. Immediately transfer them to an ice water bath to cool. Pat dry with a clean kitchen towel.

Cook Turkey Filling:

In a skillet, heat olive oil over medium heat.

Add ground turkey, ground cumin, smoked paprika, garlic powder, salt, and black pepper. Cook until the turkey is browned and fully cooked. Set aside.

Assemble Wraps:

Lay a collard green leaf flat on a clean surface.

Place a portion of the cooked turkey in the center of the leaf.

Add slices of avocado, cherry tomatoes, julienned cucumber, thinly sliced red onion, and fresh cilantro leaves.

Fold and Roll:

Fold the sides of the collard green leaf over the filling.

Starting from the bottom, roll the collard green leaf tightly to form a wrap.

Repeat with the remaining collard green leaves and filling.

Prepare Sauce:

Mix Greek yogurt or dairy-free alternatives, lime juice, honey or agave syrup, salt, and black pepper in a small bowl to create the sauce.

Serve:

Slice the Collard Green Wraps in half diagonally.

Serve the wraps with the sauce for dipping.

Enjoy:

Enjoy these Collard Green Wraps with Turkey and Avocado as a wholesome, low-carb meal that's both delicious and nutritious!

Nutrition Information (per serving): Calories: 350 Protein: 25g Carbohydrates: 20g Fat: 20g Saturated Fat: 3g Cholesterol: 50mg Sodium: 300mg Fiber: 8g Sugar: 8g

SWISS CHARD AND WHITE BEAN SOUP

Meal Description: Savor the warmth and nourishment of this hearty Swiss Chard and White Bean Soup, a comforting bowl that combines the earthy flavors of white beans with the vibrant goodness of Swiss chard. Packed with nutrients and wholesome ingredients, this soup is a delightful balance of textures and tastes. Enjoy the heartiness of white beans and the leafy goodness of Swiss chard in a flavorful broth that's perfect for a cozy meal.

Ingredients:

• 1 cup dried white beans, soaked overnight and drained (or use canned beans, rinsed and drained)

• Two tablespoons of olive oil

• One onion, finely chopped

• Three cloves garlic, minced

• Two carrots diced

• Two celery stalks, diced

• One teaspoon of dried thyme

• One bay leaf

• 6 cups vegetable or chicken broth

• One bunch of Swiss chard stems removed and leaves chopped

• Salt and black pepper to taste

• Grated Parmesan cheese for serving (optional)

• Crusty bread for serving

Instructions:

Prepare White Beans:

If using dried white beans, soak them overnight in water. Drain and rinse the beans before using. Alternatively, you can use canned white beans, rinsed and drained.

Saute Aromatics:

In a large pot, heat olive oil over medium heat.

Add finely chopped onion, minced garlic, diced carrots, and diced celery. Saute until the vegetables are softened.

Add Beans and Herbs:

Add the soaked and drained white beans to the pot.

Stir in dried thyme and add a bay leaf for flavor.

Pour in Broth:

Pour in vegetable or chicken broth, bringing the mixture to a gentle boil.

Reduce heat to low, cover, and let it simmer for 45 minutes to 1 hour until the beans are tender.

Add Swiss Chard:

Stir in chopped Swiss chard leaves, allowing them to wilt into the soup.

Season with salt and black pepper to taste.

Simmer and Serve:

Let the soup simmer for an additional 10-15 minutes, allowing the flavors to meld.

Adjust seasoning if needed.

Serve Hot:

Ladle the Swiss Chard and White Bean Soup into bowls.

Optionally, sprinkle with grated Parmesan cheese and serve with crusty bread on the side.

Enjoy:

Enjoy this wholesome and comforting soup as a nourishing meal that warms both body and soul.

Nutrition Information (per serving): Calories: 250 Protein: 12g Carbohydrates: 40g Fat: 6g Saturated Fat: 1g Cholesterol: 0mg Sodium: 800mg Fiber: 12g Sugar: 5g

WATERCRESS AND WALNUT PESTO PASTA

Meal Description: Elevate your pasta experience with this vibrant Watercress and Walnut Pesto Pasta, a dish that combines the peppery freshness of watercress with the richness of walnuts. This pesto pasta is a celebration of flavors and textures, offering a delightful balance of earthy nuts, sharp garlic, and the boldness of Parmesan cheese. Enjoy a bowl of this green goodness for a quick, nutritious, and satisfying meal.

Ingredients:

For the Watercress and Walnut Pesto:

- 2 cups fresh watercress, stems removed

- 1/2 cup walnuts

- Two cloves garlic

- 1/2 cup Parmesan cheese, grated

- 1/2 cup extra-virgin olive oil

- Salt and black pepper to taste

- Zest of 1 lemon (optional)

For the Pasta:

- 8 ounces (about 225g) of your favorite pasta

- Salt for boiling water

For Garnish (Optional):

- Additional Parmesan cheese

- Fresh watercress leaves

- Toasted walnuts

Instructions:

Prepare Watercress and Walnut Pesto:

Combine fresh watercress, walnuts, garlic, and grated Parmesan cheese in a food processor.

Pulse the ingredients until coarsely chopped.

Slowly drizzle in the extra-virgin olive oil with the food processor running until the pesto reaches a smooth consistency.

Season with salt and black pepper to taste. If desired, add the zest of one lemon for a citrusy kick.

Cook Pasta:

Bring a large pot of salted water to a boil.

Cook the pasta according to the package instructions until al dente. Reserve a cup of pasta cooking water.

Combine Pasta and Pesto:

Drain the cooked pasta and return it to the pot.

Add the watercress and walnut pesto to the pasta, tossing until the pasta is well coated. If the pesto is too thick, you can add a bit of the reserved pasta cooking water to reach your desired consistency.

Garnish and Serve:

Garnish the Watercress and Walnut Pesto Pasta with additional Parmesan cheese, fresh watercress leaves, and toasted walnuts.

Serve Hot or Cold:

Serve the pasta immediately for a comforting hot meal, or chill it in the refrigerator for a refreshing cold pasta dish.

Enjoy:

Enjoy this Watercress and Walnut Pesto Pasta as a vibrant and flavorful dish that celebrates the goodness of fresh ingredients.

Nutrition Information (per serving): Calories: 450 Protein: 12g Carbohydrates: 35g Fat: 30g Saturated Fat: 5g Cholesterol: 10mg Sodium: 200mg Fiber: 4g Sugar: 2g

ARUGULA AND TOMATO SALAD WITH BALSAMIC VINAIGRETTE

Meal Description: Delight in the simplicity and freshness of this Arugula and Tomato Salad with Balsamic Vinaigrette. This vibrant salad combines the peppery notes of arugula with the juicy sweetness of ripe tomatoes; all drizzled with a tangy balsamic vinaigrette. Enjoy this light and flavorful salad as a refreshing side dish, or add grilled chicken or shrimp for a complete, wholesome meal.

Ingredients:

For the Salad:

- 4 cups fresh arugula

- 1 pint cherry tomatoes, halved

- 1/4 cup red onion, thinly sliced

- 1/4 cup feta cheese, crumbled

- 1/4 cup pine nuts, toasted (optional)

- Fresh basil leaves for garnish

For the Balsamic Vinaigrette:

- 1/4 cup balsamic vinegar

- 1/3 cup extra-virgin olive oil

- One teaspoon of Dijon mustard

- One clove of garlic, minced

- Salt and black pepper to taste

Instructions:

Prepare Salad Ingredients:

Combine fresh arugula, halved cherry tomatoes, thinly sliced red onion, and crumbled feta cheese in a large bowl.

If using, toast the pine nuts in a dry skillet over medium heat until golden brown. Add them to the salad.

Make Balsamic Vinaigrette:

In a small bowl, whisk together balsamic vinegar, extra-virgin olive oil, Dijon mustard, minced garlic, salt, and black pepper until well combined.

Dress the Salad:

Drizzle the balsamic vinaigrette over the salad.

Toss the salad gently to ensure all ingredients are coated with the vinaigrette.

Garnish and Serve:

Garnish the Arugula and Tomato Salad with crumbled feta cheese, toasted pine nuts, and fresh basil leaves.

Serve Immediately:

Serve the salad immediately to preserve the arugula's crispness and the tomatoes' freshness.

Enjoy:

Enjoy this Arugula and Tomato Salad with Balsamic Vinaigrette as a light and refreshing dish that's perfect for any occasion.

Nutrition Information (per serving): Calories: 200 Protein: 5g Carbohydrates: 10g Fat: 16g Saturated Fat: 3.5g Cholesterol: 10mg Sodium: 200mg Fiber: 3g Sugar: 5g

BOK CHOY AND SHRIMP STIR-FRY

Meal Description: Delight in the harmony of flavors and textures with this Bok Choy and Shrimp Stir-Fry, a quick and nutritious dish that brings together the crispness of bok choy and the succulence of shrimp. Stir-fried to perfection and seasoned with a savory sauce, this meal is delicious and a wholesome option for a balanced dinner. Serve it over rice or noodles for a complete and satisfying experience.

Ingredients:

For the Stir-Fry:

- 1 pound large shrimp, peeled and deveined

- 1 pound baby bok choy, washed and halved

- One red bell pepper, thinly sliced

- One carrot, julienned

- Three cloves garlic, minced

- One tablespoon ginger, grated

- Two tablespoons of vegetable oil

- Sesame seeds for garnish (optional)

- Sliced green onions for garnish (optional)

For the Stir-Fry Sauce:

- Three tablespoons soy sauce
- Two tablespoons of oyster sauce
- One tablespoon of hoisin sauce
- One tablespoon of rice vinegar
- One teaspoon of sesame oil
- One teaspoon cornstarch
- 1/4 cup chicken or vegetable broth

Instructions:

Prepare Stir-Fry Sauce:

Whisk together soy sauce, oyster sauce, hoisin sauce, rice vinegar, sesame oil, cornstarch, and broth in a bowl. Set aside.

Stir-Fry Shrimp:

Heat one tablespoon of vegetable oil in a wok or large skillet over medium-high heat.

Add shrimp and stir-fry for 2-3 minutes until they turn pink and opaque. Remove shrimp from the wok and set aside.

Stir-Fry Vegetables:

In the same wok, add another tablespoon of vegetable oil.

Add minced garlic and grated ginger. Stir-fry for about 30 seconds until fragrant.

Add baby bok choy, red bell pepper, and julienned carrot. Stir-fry for 3-4 minutes until the vegetables are crisp-tender.

Combine Shrimp and Sauce:

Return the cooked shrimp to the wok with the vegetables.

Pour the prepared stir-fry sauce over the shrimp and vegetables.

Toss and Finish:

Toss everything together until the shrimp and vegetables are evenly coated with the sauce.

Cook for an additional 2-3 minutes until the sauce thickens.

Garnish and Serve:

Garnish the Bok Choy and Shrimp. Stir-fry with sesame seeds and sliced green onions, if desired.

Serve Hot:

Serve the stir-fry hot over rice or noodles, and enjoy the delightful combination of flavors and textures.

Nutrition Information (per serving): Calories: 300 Protein: 25g Carbohydrates: 15g Fat: 15g Saturated Fat: 2g Cholesterol: 180mg Sodium: 900mg Fiber: 5g Sugar: 5g

BEET GREENS AND GOAT CHEESE FRITTATA

Meal Description: Embark on a culinary adventure with this Beet Greens and Goat Cheese Frittata, a savory delight that transforms simple ingredients into a flavorful and satisfying dish. The earthiness of beet greens pairs perfectly with the creamy tang of goat cheese in this frittata, creating a harmonious balance of textures and tastes. Whether served for breakfast, brunch, or a light dinner, this frittata is a versatile and nutritious addition to your repertoire.

Ingredients:

- Six large eggs

- 1 cup beet greens, chopped

- 1/2 cup goat cheese, crumbled

- 1/2 cup cherry tomatoes, halved

- 1/4 cup red onion, finely chopped

- Two tablespoons fresh parsley, chopped

- One tablespoon of olive oil

- Salt and black pepper to taste

• Pinch of red pepper flakes (optional)

Instructions:

Preheat Oven:

Preheat your oven broiler.

Saute Vegetables:

In an oven-safe skillet, heat olive oil over medium heat.

Add chopped beet greens, red onion, and cherry tomatoes. Saute for 2-3 minutes until the vegetables are softened.

Whisk Eggs:

In a bowl, whisk the eggs until well beaten.

Add Eggs to Skillet:

Pour the beaten eggs over the sautéed vegetables in the skillet.

Allow the eggs to set around the edges, lifting them gently with a spatula to let the uncooked eggs flow underneath.

Add Goat Cheese and Parsley:

Sprinkle crumbled goat cheese evenly over the partially set eggs.

Add chopped fresh parsley for added flavor.

Broil the Frittata:

Place the skillet under the preheated broiler for 3-4 minutes or until the top is set and slightly golden.

Keep a close eye to prevent overcooking.

Season and Serve:

Season the Beet Greens and Goat Cheese Frittata with salt, black pepper, and a pinch of red pepper flakes if you desire a hint of spice.

Slice and Enjoy:

Carefully remove the skillet from the oven.

Slice the frittata into wedges and serve hot.

Nutrition Information (per serving): Calories: 180 Protein: 12g Carbohydrates: 4g Fat: 14g Saturated Fat: 6g Cholesterol: 320mg Sodium: 230mg Fiber: 1g Sugar: 2g

CHAPTER SIX

Recommended Fruits Recipes

Berry and Banana Smoothie Bowl

Meal Description: Indulge in a burst of freshness with this vibrant Berry and Banana Smoothie Bowl, a delightful blend of colorful berries, ripe bananas, and nutritious toppings. This smoothie bowl is a feast for the eyes and a wholesome treat for your taste buds. Customize with your favorite toppings for added texture and flavor. Whether enjoyed for breakfast or as a refreshing snack, this bowl is a nourishing and delicious way to kickstart your day.

Ingredients:

For the Smoothie Base:

• 1 cup mixed berries (strawberries, blueberries, raspberries)

• One ripe banana, frozen

• 1/2 cup Greek yogurt or dairy-free alternative

• 1/4 cup almond milk or any preferred milk

• One tablespoon of honey or maple syrup (optional, depending on sweetness preference)

• Ice cubes (optional)

For Toppings (Customizable):

• Fresh berries (sliced strawberries, blueberries, raspberries)

• Sliced banana

• Granola

• Chia seeds

- Shredded coconut
- Nut butter (almond butter, peanut butter)
- Mint leaves for garnish

Instructions:

Prepare Smoothie Base:

Combine mixed berries, frozen banana, Greek yogurt, almond milk, and honey or maple syrup in a blender.

Blend until smooth and creamy. Add ice cubes if a colder consistency is desired.

Assemble Smoothie Bowl:

Pour the smoothie base into a bowl.

Use a spatula to level the surface for even toppings.

Add Toppings:

Arrange sliced strawberries, blueberries, raspberries, and sliced bananas on top of the smoothie base.

Sprinkle granola, chia seeds, and shredded coconut for added texture.

Drizzle with your favorite nut butter for a nutty richness.

Garnish and Serve:

Garnish the Berry and Banana Smoothie Bowl with fresh mint leaves for a burst of freshness.

Optionally, add a final drizzle of honey or maple syrup.

Enjoy:

Dive into the refreshing goodness of your Berry and Banana Smoothie Bowl with a spoon and savor the delightful combination of flavors and textures.

Nutrition Information (approximate values, excluding optional toppings): Calories: 300 Protein: 12g Carbohydrates: 60g Fat: 5g Saturated Fat: 1g Cholesterol: 5mg Sodium: 60mg Fiber: 10g Sugar: 35g

FIG AND PROSCIUTTO APPETIZERS

Meal Description: Elevate your appetizer game with these Fig and Prosciutto Appetizers, a delightful combination of sweet and savory flavors that's sure to impress your guests. These bite-sized treats are visually appealing and a perfect harmony of luscious figs, creamy goat cheese, and the salty richness of prosciutto. Serve them at your next gathering for an elegant and irresistible start to your meal.

Ingredients:

- Fresh figs, halved

- Prosciutto slices, cut into strips

- Goat cheese softened

- Honey, for drizzling

- Fresh basil leaves for garnish

Instructions:

Prepare Figs:

Cut fresh figs in half lengthwise. If they have stems, you can leave the figs intact for a decorative touch.

Assemble:

Take each fig half and place a small spoonful of softened goat cheese in the center.

Wrap a strip of prosciutto around each fig half, securing the goat cheese in place.

Arrange on Serving Platter:

Arrange the prepared Fig and Prosciutto Appetizers on a serving platter.

Drizzle with Honey:

Drizzle a touch of honey over the top of each fig and prosciutto bundle for a sweet finish.

Garnish with Basil:

Garnish each appetizer with a fresh basil leaf for a burst of herbaceous aroma.

Serve:

Serve these elegant Fig and Prosciutto Appetizers at room temperature, allowing the flavors to meld.

Enjoy:

Enjoy these delightful bites that balance the sweetness of figs, goat cheese's creaminess, and prosciutto's savory richness.

Note: You can also consider adding a balsamic glaze drizzle or a sprinkle of crushed black pepper for an extra layer of flavor.

Approximate Yield: 12 appetizers

Pairing Suggestions: These appetizers pair wonderfully with a light white wine or prosecco for a sophisticated touch.

CHERRY AND ALMOND ENERGY BARS

Meal Description: Revitalize your energy with these homemade Cherry and Almond Energy Bars, packed with the goodness of dried cherries, almonds, and nutrient-rich ingredients. These bars provide a quick and convenient snack and deliver a delightful combination of sweet and nutty flavors. Whether you're on the go, hitting the gym, or need a wholesome pick-me-up, these energy bars are a delicious and nutritious choice.

Ingredients:

- 1 cup dried cherries
- 1 cup almonds, unsalted
- 1 cup rolled oats
- 1/2 cup almond butter
- 1/4 cup honey or maple syrup
- 1/4 cup chia seeds
- 1/4 cup unsweetened shredded coconut
- One teaspoon of vanilla extract
- Pinch of salt

Instructions:

Prepare a Base:

Combine dried cherries, almonds, rolled oats, chia seeds, shredded coconut, and a pinch of salt in a food processor.

Blend Ingredients:

Pulse the ingredients until they are finely chopped and well combined, creating a coarse mixture.

Add Wet Ingredients:

Add almond butter, honey or maple syrup, and vanilla extract to the mixture.

Continue to pulse until the mixture starts to come together. It should have a sticky consistency.

Press into a Pan:

Line a square or rectangular baking dish with parchment paper, leaving some overhang for easy removal.

Transfer the mixture to the dish and press it firmly and evenly using the back of a spoon or your hands.

Chill and Set:

Place the dish in the refrigerator for at least 2 hours to allow the bars to set.

Cut into Bars:

Once the Cherry and Almond Energy Bars have been developed, lift them out using the parchment paper overhang.

Place them on a cutting board and cut into bars of

your desired size.

Store:

Store the energy bars in an airtight container in the refrigerator for freshness.

Enjoy:

Grab a Cherry and Almond Energy Bar whenever you need a quick and nourishing snack to boost your energy.

Nutrition Information (per bar, approximate): Calories: 200 Protein: 6g Carbohydrates: 20g Fat: 12g Saturated Fat: 2g Cholesterol: 0mg Sodium: 20mg Fiber: 5g Sugar: 10g

PLUM AND GINGER-INFUSED WATER

Beverage Description: Quench your thirst with the refreshing and flavorful Plum and Ginger Infused Water, a delightful blend of sweet plums and zesty ginger that transforms plain Water into a hydrating sensation. This infused Water not only adds a burst of natural sweetness but also incorporates the potential health benefits of ginger. Enjoy it as a hydrating beverage on a hot day or as a unique addition to your daily water intake.

Ingredients:

• Two plums, sliced

• One small piece of fresh ginger peeled and sliced

• 1 liter (about 4 cups) of Water

• Ice cubes (optional)

• Fresh mint leaves for garnish (optional)

Instructions:

Prepare Ingredients:

Wash and slice the plums, removing the pits.

Peel and slice a small piece of fresh ginger.

Infuse Water:

In a pitcher, combine the plum slices and ginger.

Pour in the Water, ensuring that the plums and ginger are submerged.

Refrigerate:

Place the pitcher in the refrigerator and let the Plum and Ginger Infused Water chill for at least 2 hours. For a more intense flavor, you can leave it overnight.

Serve:

When ready to serve, you can strain the infused Water to remove the plum and ginger slices or leave them in for a more decorative presentation.

Add ice cubes if desired for an extra refreshing touch.

Garnish (Optional):

Garnish the infused Water with fresh mint leaves for a hint of herbal aroma and added visual appeal.

Enjoy:

Pour yourself a glass of Plum and Ginger Infused Water, sit back, and enjoy the revitalizing and naturally flavored hydration.

Note: Feel free to experiment with the intensity of flavor by adjusting the quantity of plums and ginger according to your taste preferences.

POMEGRANATE AND WALNUT CHICKEN SALAD

Meal Description: Savor the vibrant flavors and textures of this Pomegranate and Walnut Chicken Salad, a delightful combination of tender chicken, juicy pomegranate arils, crunchy walnuts, and crisp greens. Drizzled with a tangy pomegranate vinaigrette, this salad is a feast for the senses and a nourishing and satisfying meal. Enjoy it for lunch, dinner, or as a show-stopping dish at your next gathering.

Ingredients:

For the Salad:

• 2 cups cooked and shredded chicken breast

• 4 cups mixed salad greens (spinach, arugula, and mixed greens)

• 1 cup pomegranate arils

• 1/2 cup chopped walnuts, toasted

• 1/2 cup crumbled feta cheese (optional)

• One cucumber, thinly sliced

• 1/4 red onion, thinly sliced

For the Pomegranate Vinaigrette:

• 1/4 cup pomegranate juice

• Two tablespoons of red wine vinegar

• 1/3 cup extra-virgin olive oil

• One teaspoon of Dijon mustard

• One teaspoon honey

• Salt and black pepper to taste

Instructions:

Prepare Chicken:

Cook chicken breasts by baking, grilling, or poaching. Shred the cooked chicken into bite-sized pieces.

Prepare Salad Greens:

In a large bowl, combine the mixed salad greens, shredded chicken, pomegranate arils, chopped toasted walnuts, crumbled feta cheese (if using), cucumber slices, and thinly sliced red onion.

Make Pomegranate Vinaigrette:

Whisk together pomegranate juice, red wine vinegar, extra-virgin olive oil, Dijon mustard, honey, salt, and black pepper in a small bowl. Adjust the seasoning to taste.

Toss Salad with Dressing:

Drizzle the Pomegranate Vinaigrette over the salad.

Gently toss the salad to ensure it is even coated with the dressing.

Serve:

Transfer the salad to individual plates or a serving platter.

Garnish (Optional):

Garnish the Pomegranate and Walnut Chicken Salad with additional pomegranate arils, chopped walnuts, and crumbled feta cheese if desired.

Enjoy:

Dive into the delicious medley of flavors and textures in this Pomegranate and Walnut Chicken Salad. Serve immediately and enjoy!

Nutrition Information (per serving, approximate): Calories: 400 Protein: 25g Carbohydrates: 20g Fat: 25g Saturated Fat: 4g Cholesterol: 60mg Sodium: 300mg Fiber: 5g Sugar: 10g

PEACH AND RASPBERRY PARFAIT

Dessert Description: Indulge in the sweetness of summer with this Peach and Raspberry Parfait, a delightful layered dessert that combines the juicy goodness of ripe peaches with the tartness of fresh raspberries. Each spoonful is a symphony of flavors and textures, enhanced by the creamy richness of yogurt and the crunch of granola. Whether served as a light dessert or a refreshing snack, this parfait celebrates celebrates seasonal fruits and treats for your taste buds.

Ingredients:

• Two ripe peaches, peeled and diced

• 1 cup fresh raspberries

• 2 cups Greek yogurt or your favorite yogurt

• 1/2 cup granola

• Two tablespoons honey or maple syrup (optional)

• Fresh mint leaves for garnish (optional)

Instructions:

Prepare Fruits:

Peel and dice the ripe peaches.

Rinse the fresh raspberries.

Assemble Parfait:

Start by layering a spoonful of Greek yogurt at the bottom of serving glasses or bowls.

Add a layer of diced peaches on top of the yogurt.

Follow with a layer of fresh raspberries.

Repeat the layers until the glasses are filled, finishing with a dollop of yogurt on the top.

Add Granola:

Sprinkle granola over the yogurt layer for a crunchy texture.

Drizzle with Honey (Optional):

If desired, drizzle honey or maple syrup over the top for added sweetness.

Garnish (Optional):

Garnish the Peach and Raspberry Parfait with fresh mint leaves for a burst of herbal aroma and visual appeal.

Serve Immediately:

Serve the parfait immediately to enjoy the contrast of creamy yogurt, juicy fruits, and crunchy granola.

Enjoy:

Delight in the Peach and Raspberry Parfait is a refreshing and satisfying dessert that captures the essence of summer.

Nutrition Information (per serving, approximate): Calories: 300 Protein: 15g Carbohydrates: 40g Fat: 8g Saturated Fat: 2g Cholesterol: 10mg Sodium: 80mg Fiber: 6g Sugar: 20g

GRAPEFRUIT AND AVOCADO SALAD

Salad Description: Elevate your salad experience with this refreshing and vibrant Grapefruit and Avocado Salad. The zesty citrus of grapefruit combines perfectly with the creamy texture of avocado, creating a delightful medley of flavors. Tossed with mixed greens and drizzled with a citrusy vinaigrette, this salad is a feast for the senses and a nutritious addition to your meal. Enjoy it as a light lunch or a refreshing side dish.

Ingredients:

For the Salad:

- Two pink grapefruits, segmented

- Two ripe avocados, sliced

- 6 cups mixed salad greens (arugula, spinach, and watercress)

- 1/4 cup red onion, thinly sliced

- 1/4 cup fresh mint leaves, torn

- 1/4 cup crumbled feta cheese (optional)

For the Citrus Vinaigrette:

- 1/4 cup fresh grapefruit juice

- Two tablespoons of fresh orange juice

- Three tablespoons extra-virgin olive oil
- One teaspoon of honey or maple syrup
- Salt and black pepper to taste

Instructions:

Prepare Grapefruit Segments:

Peel and segment the pink grapefruits over a bowl to catch any juice.

Make Citrus Vinaigrette:

In a small bowl, whisk together fresh grapefruit juice, fresh orange juice, extra-virgin olive oil, honey or maple syrup, salt, and black pepper to create the Citrus Vinaigrette.

Assemble Salad:

Combine the mixed salad greens, grapefruit segments, sliced ripe avocados, thinly sliced red onion, and torn fresh mint leaves in a large salad bowl.

If using, sprinkle crumbled feta cheese over the salad.

Drizzle with Citrus Vinaigrette:

Drizzle the Citrus Vinaigrette over the salad.

Toss Gently:

Toss the salad gently to ensure all ingredients are well coated with the vinaigrette.

Serve:

Transfer the Grapefruit and Avocado Salad to individual plates or a serving platter.

Garnish (Optional):

Garnish the salad with additional mint leaves and a sprinkle of black pepper if desired.

Enjoy:

Enjoy this refreshing and nutritious Grapefruit and Avocado Salad as a light and flavorful addition to your meal.

Nutrition Information (per serving, approximate): Calories: 250 Protein: 4g Carbohydrates: 20g Fat: 18g Saturated Fat: 3g Cholesterol: 5mg Sodium: 100mg Fiber: 8g Sugar: 10g

PAPAYA AND LIME SORBET

Dessert Description: Cool down with the tropical goodness of Papaya and Lime Sorbet, a refreshing frozen treat that brings together the natural sweetness of papaya with a zingy burst of lime. This sorbet is a delightful palate cleanser and a guilt-free dessert option. Whether enjoyed on a hot summer day or as a light and fruity finale to a meal, this sorbet is sure to become a favorite.

Ingredients:

• 3 cups ripe papaya, peeled, seeded, and cubed

• 1/2 cup fresh lime juice (about four limes)

• 1/2 cup water

• 1/2 cup granulated sugar

• Zest of 1 lime (for garnish, optional)

• Mint leaves for garnish (optional)

Instructions:

Prepare Papaya:

Peel, seed, and cube the ripe papaya.

Make Simple Syrup:

In a small saucepan, combine Water and

granulated sugar. Heat over medium heat, stirring occasionally, until the sugar is completely dissolved. Allow the simple syrup to cool.

Blend Ingredients:

Combine the cubed papaya, fresh lime juice, and the cooled simple syrup in a blender.

Blend until the mixture is smooth and well combined.

Strain (Optional):

If desired, strain the sorbet mixture using a fine mesh sieve to remove any pulp. This step is optional, depending on your preference for texture.

Chill:

Transfer the sorbet mixture to a bowl, cover, and refrigerate for at least 2 hours or until thoroughly chilled.

Freeze:

Once chilled, transfer the mixture to an ice cream maker and churn according to the manufacturer's instructions until it reaches a sorbet consistency.

If you don't have an ice cream maker, pour the mixture into a shallow dish and freeze. Every 30 minutes, stir with a fork to break up ice crystals until the sorbet reaches the desired consistency.

Serve:

Scoop the Papaya and Lime Sorbet into bowls or cones.

Garnish (Optional):

Garnish with lime zest and fresh mint leaves for a burst of color and aroma.

Enjoy:

Enjoy the tropical delight of Papaya and Lime Sorbet as a refreshing and guilt-free dessert.

Note: This sorbet can be stored in an airtight container in the freezer for several weeks. Allow it to soften for a few minutes before serving if frozen solid.

KIWI AND STRAWBERRY SALAD WITH MINT

Salad Description: Delight in the vibrant combination of flavors and colors with this Kiwi and Strawberry Salad with Mint. Fresh kiwi and ripe strawberries come together with the invigorating aroma of mint to create a refreshing and wholesome salad. Drizzled with a honey-lime dressing, this salad perfectly balances sweet and tart, making it a delightful addition to any meal or a light and fruity snack.

Ingredients:

For the Salad:

• Four kiwis, peeled and sliced

• 2 cups fresh strawberries, hulled and halved

• One tablespoon of of fresh mint leaves, finely chopped

• One tablespoon honey (optional for drizzling)

For the Honey-Lime Dressing:

• Two tablespoons of fresh lime juice

• One tablespoon honey

• One tablespoon extra-virgin olive oil

Instructions:

Prepare Kiwis and Strawberries:

Peel and slice the kiwis into rounds or halves.

Hull the strawberries and cut them into halves.

Make Honey-Lime Dressing:

Whisk together fresh lime juice, honey, and extra-virgin olive oil in a small bowl to create the Honey-Lime Dressing.

Assemble Salad:

In a serving bowl, combine the sliced kiwis and halved strawberries.

Sprinkle the finely chopped mint leaves over the fruits.

Drizzle with Dressing:

Drizzle the Honey-Lime Dressing over the kiwi and strawberry mixture.

If desired, drizzle an additional tablespoon of honey over the top for extra sweetness.

Gently Toss:

Gently toss the salad to ensure it is even coated with the dressing.

Chill (Optional):

If time allows, refrigerate the salad for 15-30 minutes to let the flavors meld and the salad chill.

Serve:

Serve the Kiwi and Strawberry Salad with Mint in individual bowls or as a colorful side dish.

Garnish (Optional):

Garnish with additional mint leaves for a fresh and aromatic touch.

Enjoy:

Enjoy this light and fruity Kiwi and Strawberry Salad with Mint as a refreshing treat.

Note: Feel free to customize the salad by adding a handful of blueberries or a sprinkle of chopped nuts for additional texture and flavor.

CHAPTER SEVEN

Recommended Nuts
and Seeds Recipes

Walnut-Crusted Salmon

Main Course Description: Elevate your salmon game with this Walnut-Crusted Salmon recipe, where walnuts' rich and nutty flavor forms a deliciously crunchy crust for the tender salmon fillets. Paired with a hint of lemon and herbs, this dish perfectly balances textures and tastes. Serve it as a centerpiece for a wholesome dinner, and delight in the fusion of omega-3-rich salmon and heart-healthy walnuts.

Ingredients:

- Four salmon fillets (6 ounces each), skin-on or skinless

- 1 cup walnuts, finely chopped

- Two tablespoons fresh parsley, chopped

- Two tablespoons of grated Parmesan cheese

- One tablespoon of Dijon mustard

- One tablespoon of lemon juice

- Two tablespoons of olive oil

- Salt and black pepper to taste

- Lemon wedges for serving

- Fresh parsley for garnish (optional)

Instructions:

Preheat Oven:

Preheat your oven to 400°F (200°C).

Prepare Walnut Crust Mixture:

Combine finely chopped walnuts, chopped fresh parsley, grated Parmesan cheese, Dijon mustard, lemon juice, and olive oil in a bowl. Mix well to create the walnut crust mixture.

Season Salmon:

Pat the salmon fillets dry with paper towels.

Season both sides of the salmon fillet with salt and black pepper to taste.

Coat with Walnut Mixture:

Place the salmon fillets on a baking sheet lined with parchment paper.

Coat the top side of each salmon fillet with the walnut crust mixture, pressing it gently to adhere.

Bake:

Bake in the preheated oven for 12-15 minutes or until the salmon is cooked through and the walnut crust is golden brown.

Broil (Optional):

If desired, you can broil the salmon for 1-2 minutes to crispen the walnut crust further.

Serve:

Carefully transfer the Walnut-Crusted Salmon to serving plates.

Garnish (Optional):

Garnish with fresh parsley and serve with lemon wedges on the side.

Enjoy:

Enjoy the Walnut-Crusted Salmon as a flavorful

and nutritious main course.

Note: This recipe works well with both skin-on and skinless salmon fillets. Adjust the cooking time based on the thickness of your salmon fillets to ensure they are cooked to perfection.

ALMOND AND DATE PROTEIN BALLS

Snack Description: Energize your day with these Almond and Date Protein Balls, a wholesome and delicious snack that combines the natural sweetness of dates with the nutty goodness of almonds. Packed with protein and fiber, these no-bake bites are perfect for a quick pick-me-up, post-workout snack, or a guilt-free treat. Make a batch and keep them on hand for a convenient and nutritious bite whenever you need it.

Ingredients:

• 1 cup pitted dates, soaked in warm water for 10 minutes

• 1 cup almonds

• Two tablespoons of almond butter

• 1/4 cup protein powder (vanilla or chocolate flavor)

• 1/2 teaspoon vanilla extract

• Pinch of salt

• Shredded coconut or crushed almonds for coating (optional)

Instructions:

Soak Dates:

Place pitted dates in warm water and let them soak

for about 10 minutes to soften.

Prepare Almonds:

In a food processor, pulse almonds until they are finely ground. Some small almond pieces for texture are okay.

Blend Ingredients:

Drain the soaked dates and add them to the food processor with the ground almonds.

Add almond butter, protein powder, vanilla extract, and a pinch of salt.

Blend the mixture until it forms a sticky dough.

Shape into Balls:

With slightly damp hands, roll portions of the mixture into bite-sized balls.

Optional Coating:

If desired, roll the protein balls in shredded coconut or crushed almonds for an extra layer of texture.

Chill:

Place the Almond and Date Protein Balls in the refrigerator for at least 30 minutes to firm up.

Store:

Store the protein balls in an airtight container in the fridge for a longer shelf life.

Enjoy:

Grab some Almond and Date Protein Balls for a nutritious and satisfying snack.

Note: Feel free to customize by adding chia seeds, flaxseeds, or a dash of cinnamon for added flavor and nutritional benefits. Adjust the quantity of almond butter or protein powder to achieve the desired texture.

PISTACHIO-CRUSTED CHICKEN TENDERS

Main Course Description: Add a delightful crunch to your chicken tenders with this Pistachio-Crusted Chicken Tenders recipe. The nutty flavor of pistachios combines with a savory blend of herbs and spices, creating a flavorful and satisfying dish. These crispy chicken tenders are sure to become a favorite, perfect for a family-friendly dinner or a crowd-pleasing appetizer. Serve them with your favorite dipping sauce for an extra burst of flavor.

Ingredients:

• 1 pound chicken tenders

• 1 cup shelled pistachios, finely chopped

• 1/2 cup breadcrumbs (optional for additional crispiness)

• One teaspoon of garlic powder

• One teaspoon of onion powder

• One teaspoon paprika

• 1/2 teaspoon dried thyme

• Salt and black pepper to taste

• Two eggs, beaten

• Cooking spray or olive oil for baking

Instructions:

Preheat Oven:

Preheat your oven to 400°F (200°C). Line a baking sheet with parchment paper.

Prepare Pistachios:

Finely chop the shelled pistachios in a food processor until they resemble breadcrumbs. Transfer them to a shallow bowl.

Add Seasonings:

Add garlic powder, onion powder, paprika, dried thyme, salt, and black pepper to the chopped pistachios. Mix well to combine.

Coat Chicken Tenders:

Dip each chicken tender into the beaten eggs, ensuring it's fully coated.

Roll the egg-coated chicken tender in the pistachio and spice mixture, pressing gently to adhere to the coating.

You can roll the chicken tender in breadcrumbs after coating it with the pistachio mixture for an extra crispy texture.

Place on Baking Sheet:

Arrange the coated chicken tenders on the prepared baking sheet.

Bake:

Lightly spray the chicken tenders with cooking spray or drizzle with olive oil for added crispiness.

Bake in the preheated oven for 15-18 minutes or until the chicken is cooked through and the crust is golden brown.

Serve:

Transfer the Pistachio-Crusted Chicken Tenders to a serving platter.

Dipping Sauce (Optional):

Serve with your favorite dipping sauce, such as honey mustard, yogurt-based sauce, or a tangy barbecue sauce.

Enjoy:

Enjoy these delicious and nutty Pistachio-Crusted Chicken Tenders as a wholesome and flavorful meal.

Note: Adjust the seasoning according to your taste preferences. If you prefer a more intense flavor, you can add a pinch of cayenne pepper or smoked paprika to the pistachio mixture.

SUNFLOWER SEED PESTO PASTA

Main Course Description: Experience a twist on classic pesto with this Sunflower Seed Pesto Pasta, where sunflower seeds' rich and nutty flavor takes center stage. This vibrant and flavorful pasta dish is a delightful alternative to traditional pesto, offering a nut-free option for those with allergies. Toss it with your favorite pasta for a quick and satisfying meal that brings together the goodness of fresh herbs, garlic, Parmesan, and sunflower seeds.

Ingredients:

For the Sunflower Seed Pesto:

• 1 cup fresh basil leaves, packed

• 1/2 cup sunflower seeds, toasted

• 1/2 cup grated Parmesan cheese

• Two cloves garlic

• 1/2 cup extra-virgin olive oil

• Salt and black pepper to taste

• Juice of half a lemon

For the Pasta:

• 12 ounces (340g) of your favorite pasta (spaghetti,

penne, or fusilli)

- Cherry tomatoes, halved (for garnish)

- Fresh basil leaves (for garnish)

- Grated Parmesan cheese (for serving)

Instructions:

Toast Sunflower Seeds:

Over medium heat, toast the sunflower seeds in a dry skillet until they become golden brown and fragrant. Stir frequently to prevent burning. Allow them to cool.

Cook Pasta:

Cook the pasta according to the package instructions until al dente. Drain and set aside.

Prepare Sunflower Seed Pesto:

Combine fresh basil leaves, toasted sunflower seeds, grated Parmesan cheese, garlic cloves, salt, and black pepper in a food processor.

Pulse the ingredients while slowly pouring in the olive oil until the mixture forms a smooth and well-combined pesto.

Squeeze in the juice of half a lemon and pulse once more to incorporate.

Toss Pasta with Pesto:

In a large bowl, toss the cooked pasta with the sunflower seed pesto until the pasta is evenly coated.

Garnish:

Garnish the Sunflower Seed Pesto Pasta with

halved cherry tomatoes and fresh basil leaves.

Serve:

Divide the pasta into individual plates, sprinkle with additional grated Parmesan cheese if desired, and serve.

Enjoy:

Enjoy this delightful Sunflower Seed Pesto Pasta as a flavorful and nutty twist on a classic dish.

Note: Feel free to customize the pesto by adding a handful of spinach or arugula for extra freshness and nutritional benefits. Adjust the consistency of the pesto by adding more olive oil if needed.

PUMPKIN SEED-CRUSTED TOFU STIR-FRY

Main Course Description: Transform your tofu stir-fry with a crunchy twist using this Pumpkin Seed-Crusted Tofu recipe. Coated in a flavorful blend of pumpkin seeds and spices, the tofu becomes irresistibly crispy, adding a delightful texture to the stir-fry. Paired with a medley of colorful vegetables and a savory sauce, this dish is a celebration of plant-based goodness and exciting flavors.

Ingredients:

For the Pumpkin Seed-Crusted Tofu:

• One block of extra-firm tofu pressed and cut into cubes

• 1 cup raw pumpkin seeds

• One teaspoon of smoked paprika

• 1/2 teaspoon cumin

• 1/2 teaspoon garlic powder

• Salt and black pepper to taste

• Two tablespoons of olive oil

For the Stir-Fry:

• 2 cups broccoli florets

- One bell pepper, thinly sliced
- One carrot, julienned
- 1 cup snap peas, ends trimmed
- Three green onions, sliced
- Two tablespoons of soy sauce
- One tablespoon of sesame oil
- One tablespoon of rice vinegar
- One tablespoon of maple syrup or agave nectar
- Sesame seeds for garnish
- Cooked brown rice or noodles (optional for serving)

Instructions:

Prepare Pumpkin Seed Coating:

Combine raw pumpkin seeds, smoked paprika, cumin, garlic powder, salt, and black pepper in a food processor. Pulse until the pumpkin seeds are finely ground.

Coat Tofu:

Press the tofu to remove excess water, then cut it into cubes.

Coat each tofu cube in the pumpkin seed mixture, pressing the coating gently to adhere.

Cook Pumpkin Seed-Crusted Tofu:

In a large skillet, heat olive oil over medium heat.

Add the pumpkin seed-crusted tofu cubes and cook until all sides are golden brown and crispy. Set aside.

Prepare Stir-Fry Sauce:

Whisk together soy sauce, sesame oil, rice vinegar, maple syrup, or agave nectar in a small bowl to create the stir-fry sauce. Set aside.

Stir-Fry Vegetables:

In the same skillet, stir-fry broccoli, bell pepper, carrot, snap peas, and green onions until they are tender-crisp.

Combine Tofu and Vegetables:

Add the cooked pumpkin seed-crusted tofu to the vegetables in the skillet.

Pour the stir-fry sauce over the tofu and vegetables, tossing to coat evenly.

Serve:

Serve the Pumpkin Seed-Crusted Tofu Stir-Fry over cooked brown rice or noodles if desired.

Garnish:

Garnish with sesame seeds for an extra crunch.

Enjoy:

Enjoy this flavorful and protein-packed Pumpkin Seed-Crusted Tofu Stir-Fry as a satisfying plant-based meal.

Note: Feel free to customize the stir-fry by adding your favorite vegetables or adjusting the level of spice in the pumpkin seed coating.

HAZELNUT AND BERRY SALAD WITH BALSAMIC DRESSING

Salad Description: Indulge in the delightful combination of sweet and savory with this Hazelnut and Berry Salad featuring a medley of fresh berries, crunchy hazelnuts, and a tangy balsamic dressing. This vibrant and nutritious salad is a celebration of flavors and textures, making it a perfect addition to any meal or a light and refreshing standalone dish.

Ingredients:

For the Salad:

• 6 cups mixed salad greens (arugula, spinach, and mesclun mix)

• 1 cup strawberries, hulled and sliced

• 1/2 cup blueberries

• 1/2 cup raspberries

• 1/2 cup blackberries

• 1/2 cup crumbled feta cheese or goat cheese

- 1/2 cup hazelnuts, toasted and chopped

For the Balsamic Dressing:

- 1/4 cup balsamic vinegar

- 1/3 cup extra-virgin olive oil

- One tablespoon of Dijon mustard

- One tablespoon of honey or maple syrup

- Salt and black pepper to taste

Instructions:

Prepare Salad Greens:

Combine the mixed salad greens in a large salad bowl, ensuring they are well-washed and dried.

Add Berries and Cheese:

Add sliced strawberries, blueberries, raspberries, blackberries, and crumbled feta or goat cheese to the salad.

Toast Hazelnuts:

In a dry skillet over medium heat, toast the hazelnuts until they become fragrant and lightly browned. Allow them to cool, then chop coarsely.

Sprinkle Hazelnuts:

Sprinkle the toasted and chopped hazelnuts over the salad for added crunch.

Prepare Balsamic Dressing:

In a small bowl, whisk together balsamic vinegar, extra-virgin olive oil, Dijon mustard, honey or maple syrup, salt, and black pepper until well combined.

Drizzle Dressing:

Drizzle the balsamic dressing over the salad, starting with a small amount and adding more as needed.

Toss Gently:

Gently toss the salad to ensure all ingredients are evenly coated with the dressing.

Serve:

Transfer the Hazelnut and Berry Salad to individual plates or a serving platter.

Enjoy:

Enjoy this vibrant and flavorful salad as a refreshing side dish or a light and nutritious main course.

Note: Feel free to customize the salad by adding avocado slices or swapping out the type of berries based on seasonal availability. Adjust the sweetness of the dressing according to your taste preferences.

CHIA SEED BREAKFAST PUDDING

Breakfast Description: Start your day on a nutritious note with this Chia Seed Breakfast Pudding. Packed with fiber, omega-3 fatty acids, and antioxidants, this pudding is delicious and a healthy way to fuel your morning. Customize it with your favorite toppings, such as fresh fruits, nuts, or a drizzle of honey, for a breakfast that's as visually appealing as it is satisfying.

Ingredients:

• 1/4 cup chia seeds

• 1 cup unsweetened almond milk (or your preferred milk)

• One tablespoon of maple syrup or honey

• 1/2 teaspoon vanilla extract

• Fresh fruits (berries, sliced banana, etc.) for topping

• Nuts or seeds (almonds, walnuts, sunflower seeds, etc.) for topping

• Honey or maple syrup for drizzling (optional)

Instructions:

Mix Chia Seeds and Liquid:

Combine chia seeds, almond milk, maple syrup or honey, and vanilla extract in a bowl or jar. Stir well to combine.

Let it Set:

Cover the bowl or jar and refrigerate the mixture for at least 4 hours or preferably overnight. This allows the chia seeds to absorb the liquid and create a pudding-like consistency.

Stir Again (Optional):

After the initial setting time, you can give the mixture a stir to ensure that the chia seeds are evenly distributed.

Top with Fresh Fruits and Nuts:

When ready to serve, top the Chia Seed Breakfast Pudding with your favorite fresh fruits (berries, sliced banana, etc.) and a sprinkle of nuts or seeds.

Drizzle with Honey or Maple Syrup (Optional):

You can drizzle honey or maple syrup over the top for added sweetness.

Serve and Enjoy:

Spoon the delicious Chia Seed Breakfast Pudding into a bowl, or enjoy it directly from the jar. It's a nutritious and satisfying way to start your day.

Note: Feel free to experiment with different milk alternatives, such as coconut milk, oat milk, or dairy milk, based on your preferences. Customize the toppings to suit your taste, and enjoy the versatility of this wholesome breakfast option.

SESAME-CRUSTED AHI TUNA

Main Course Description: Elevate your seafood experience with this Sesame-Crusted Ahi Tuna recipe. The combination of sesame seeds, spices, and fresh tuna creates a flavorful crust with a perfectly seared exterior and a rare, tender center. Serve it with a zesty dipping sauce for a restaurant-worthy dish that's both delicious and visually stunning.

Ingredients:

For the Sesame-Crusted Ahi Tuna:

• Two ahi tuna steaks, sushi-grade (about 6-8 ounces each)

• 1/4 cup white sesame seeds

• 1/4 cup black sesame seeds

• One teaspoon of ground coriander

• One teaspoon of ground cumin

• Salt and black pepper to taste

• Two tablespoons of soy sauce

• One tablespoon of sesame oil

• One tablespoon vegetable oil (for searing)

For the Dipping Sauce:

- 1/4 cup soy sauce

- One tablespoon of rice vinegar

- One tablespoon of honey or maple syrup

- One teaspoon of grated fresh ginger

- One teaspoon of sesame oil

- Optional: sliced green onions and sesame seeds for garnish

Instructions:

Prepare Tuna Steaks:

Pat the ahi tuna steaks dry with paper towels.

Combine Sesame Seeds and Spices:

Combine white sesame seeds, black sesame seeds, ground coriander, ground cumin, salt, and black pepper in a shallow dish.

Coat Tuna Steaks:

Brush the ahi tuna steaks with soy sauce and sesame oil, ensuring they are well coated.

Press the tuna steaks into the sesame seed and spice mixture, coating all sides evenly. Gently press the sesame seeds onto the tuna to adhere.

Sear Tuna Steaks:

Heat vegetable oil in a skillet or pan over high heat.

Sear the sesame-crusted tuna steaks for about 1-2 minutes on each side or until the sesame crust is golden brown, leaving the center rare.

Slice and Arrange:

Remove the tuna steaks from the pan and let them

rest for a minute.

Slice the tuna into thin, even slices.

Prepare Dipping Sauce:

Whisk together soy sauce, rice vinegar, honey or maple syrup, grated fresh ginger, and sesame oil in a small bowl to create the dipping sauce.

Serve:

Arrange the sesame-crusted ahi tuna slices on a serving platter.

Drizzle the dipping sauce over the tuna.

Garnish (Optional):

Garnish with sliced green onions and additional sesame seeds if desired.

Enjoy:

Serve immediately and enjoy the Sesame-Crusted Ahi Tuna with its flavorful crust and a hint of rare freshness.

Note: Adjust the cooking time based on your preference for the tuna's doneness. If you prefer a fully cooked tuna, sear for an additional minute on each side.

CONCLUSION

In the realm of nutritional science, the Blood Type Diet, with its tailored approach based on blood type O, has stirred curiosity and debate. While the concept of associating specific dietary recommendations with blood type adds an intriguing dimension to personalized nutrition, it is important to approach such claims with a discerning eye.

The notion that blood type O is linked to the traits of ancient hunter-gatherer societies, influencing optimal dietary choices, remains controversial within the scientific community. Critics argue that the diet lacks robust scientific evidence and overlooks the complexity of individual nutritional needs. Nutrition is a multifaceted field, influenced by factors such as genetics, lifestyle, and overall health, and the one-size-fits-all approach advocated by the Blood Type Diet may need to address the diversity of human physiology adequately.

Scientifically, there is a consensus that nutritional recommendations should be based on comprehensive evidence rather than a singular factor like blood type. Personalized dietary advice, taking into account an individual's health status, preferences, and cultural considerations, is more likely to contribute to long-term well-being.

www.ingramcontent.com/pod-product-compliance
Lightning Source LLC
Chambersburg PA
CBHW050727260726

48661CB00001B/102